BREAST CANCER. SERIOUSLY?

HOT CHICKS GET CANCER TOO
Going From
Hot to Not
To Loving Me a Lot

Written and Illustrated
By Pat Sullivan

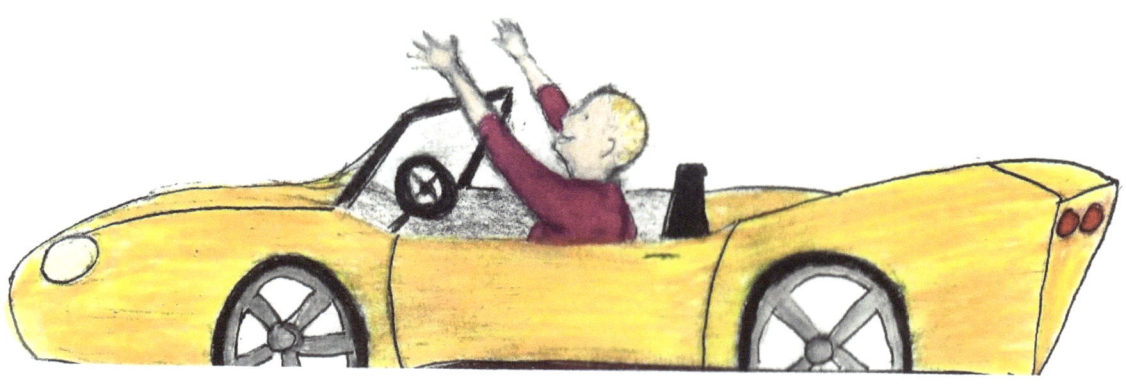

Copyright © 2021 Pat Sullivan

All rights reserved. No part of this publication may be reproduced, distributed or transmitted in any form, or by any means, or stored in a database or retrieval system without the prior written permission of the copyright holder.

Connect with the author using #breastcancerseriously

ISBN: 979-8-68107-923-1

This book is dedicated to –

All those whose lives have been affected by cancer.

God, who pursued my heart and let me know everything was going to be OK.

Eric, whom I love dearly.

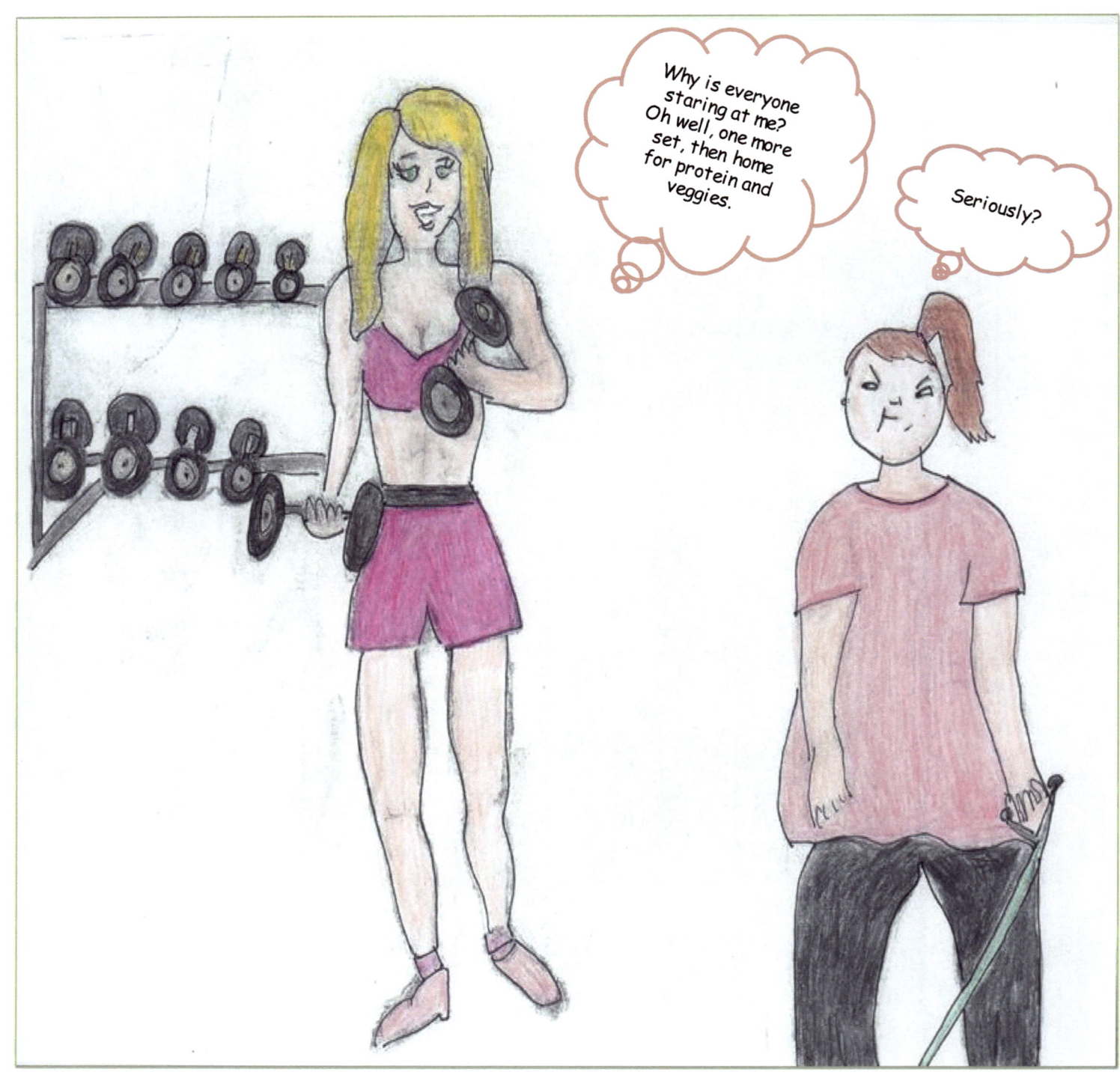

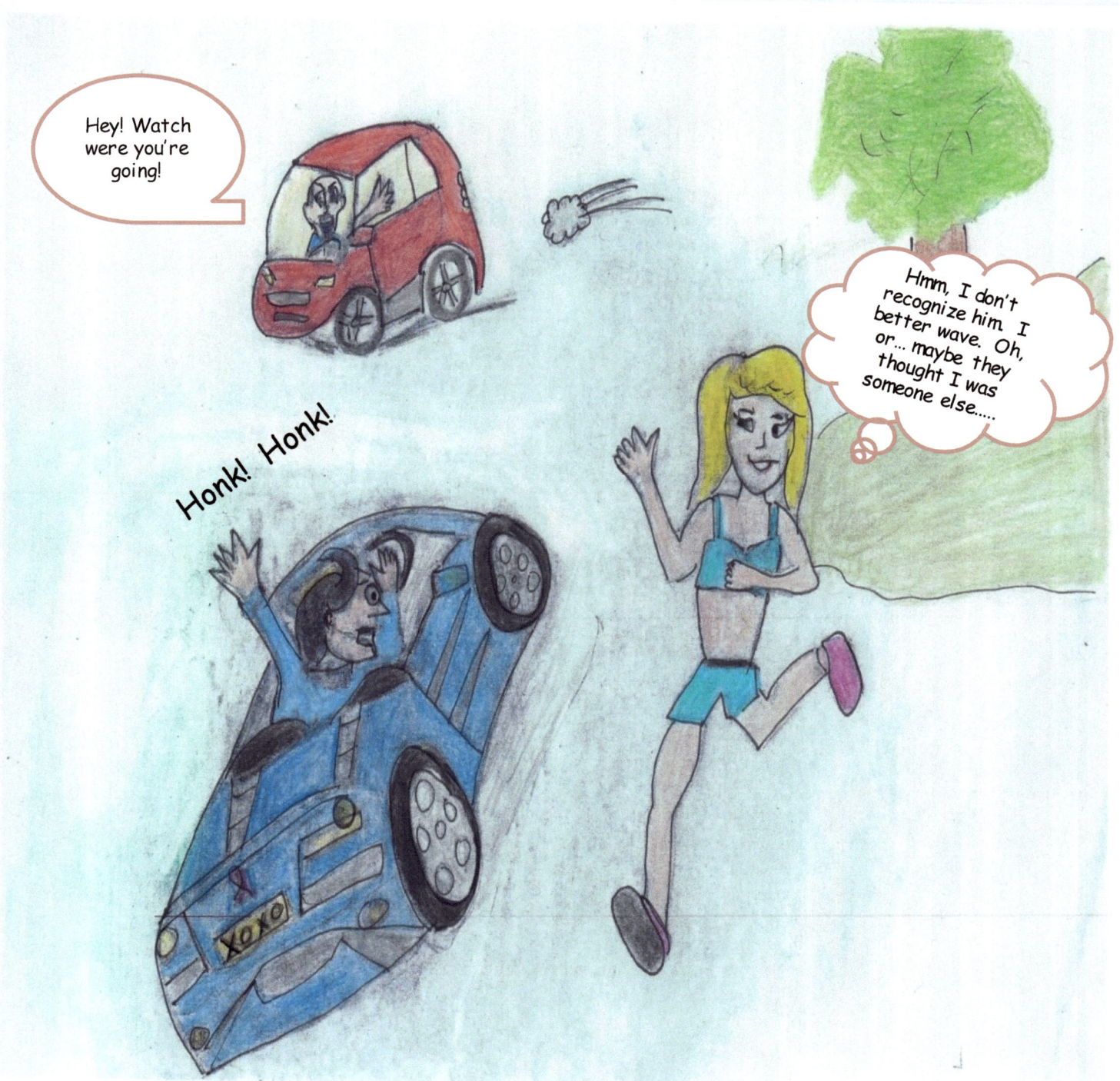

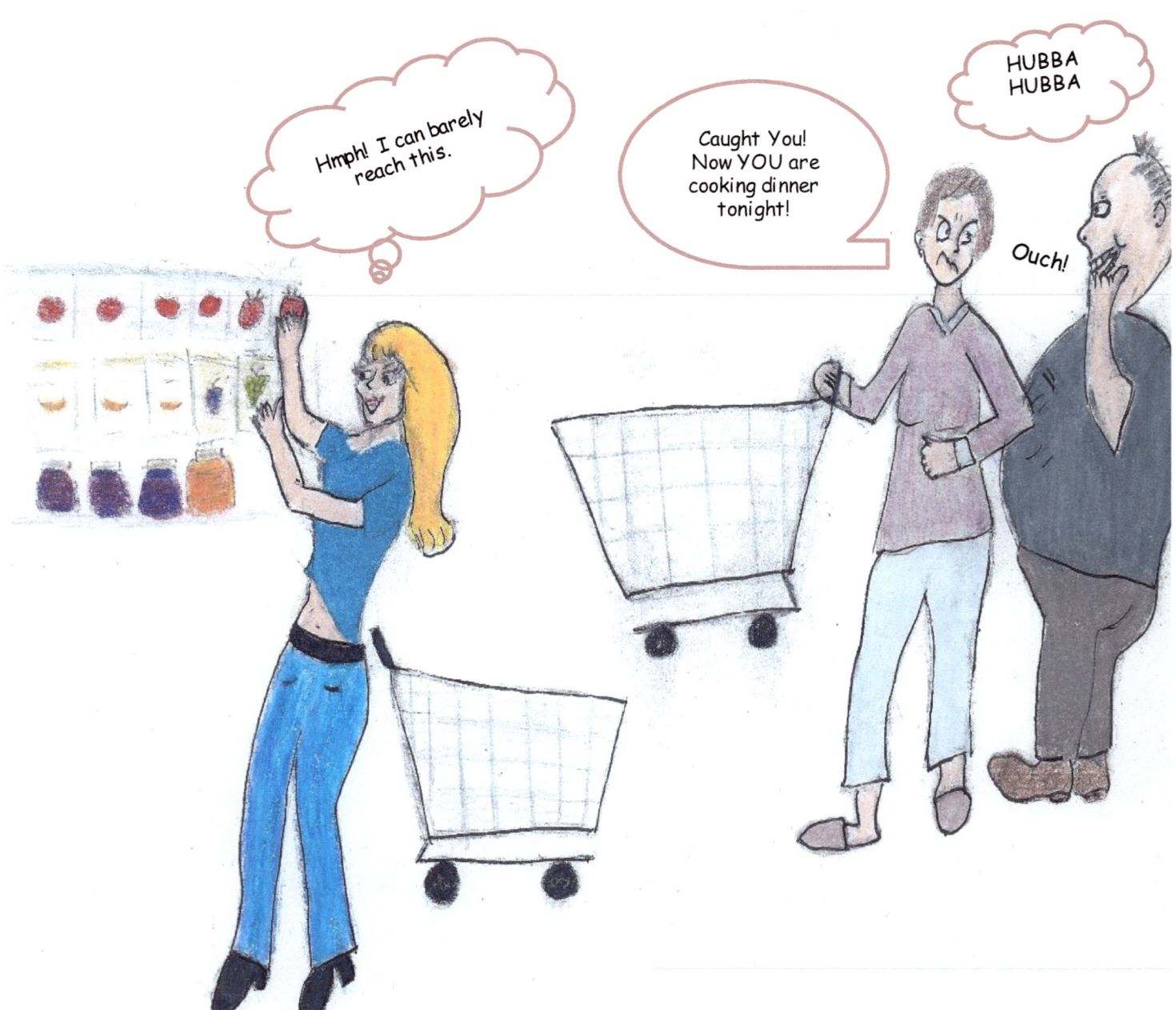

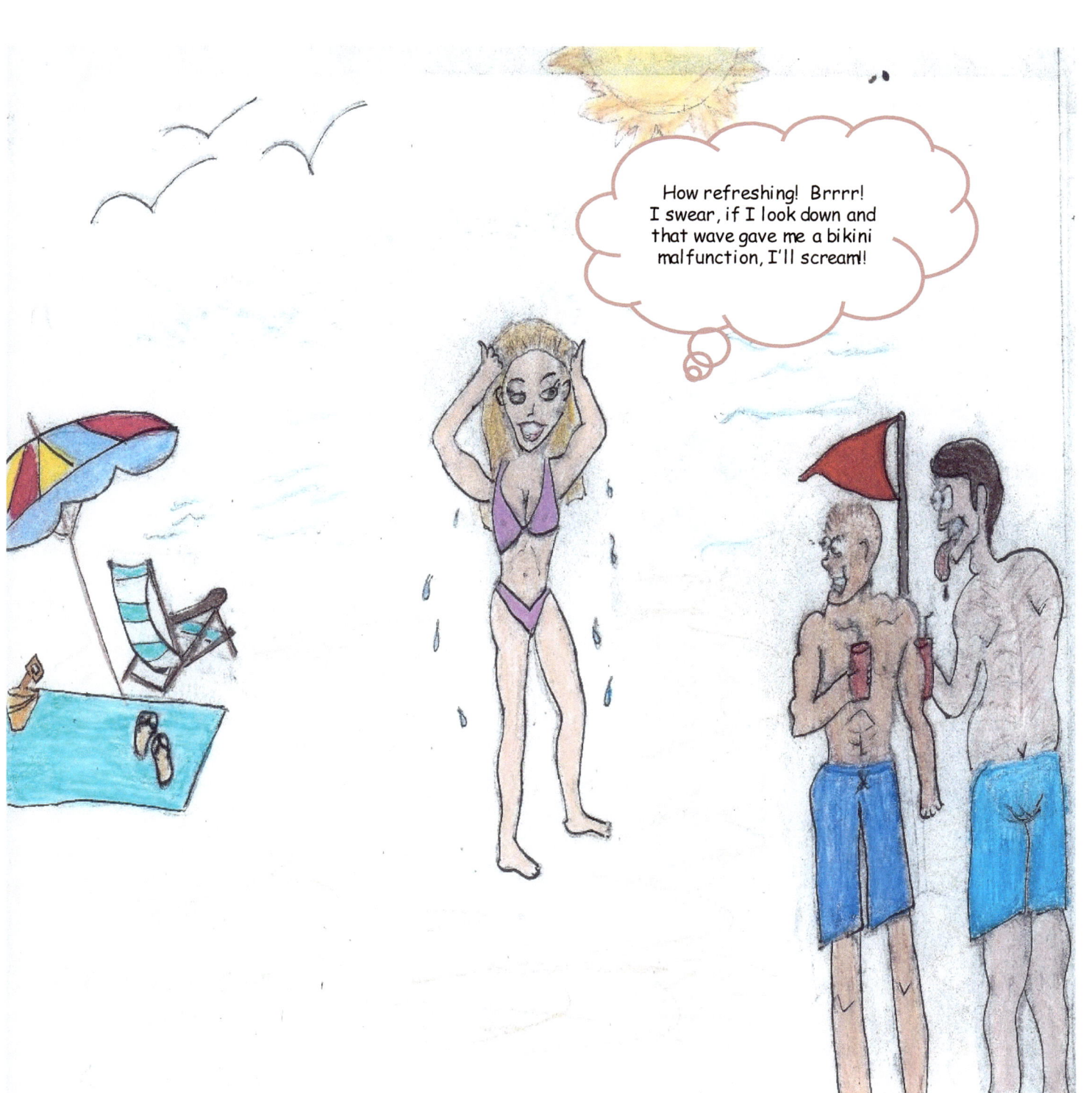

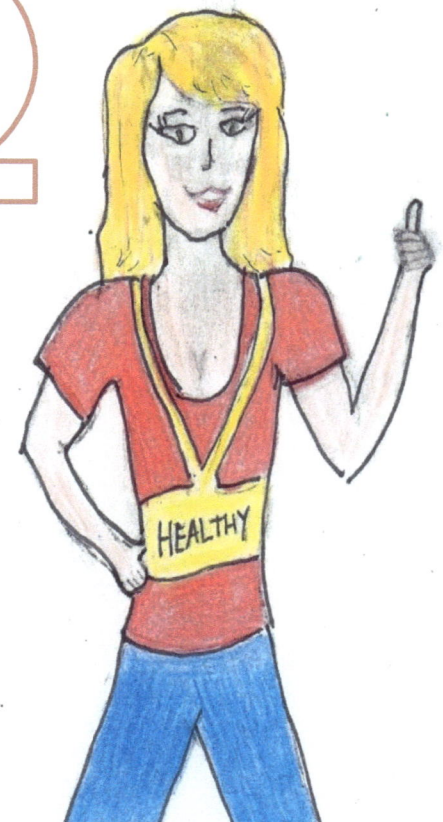

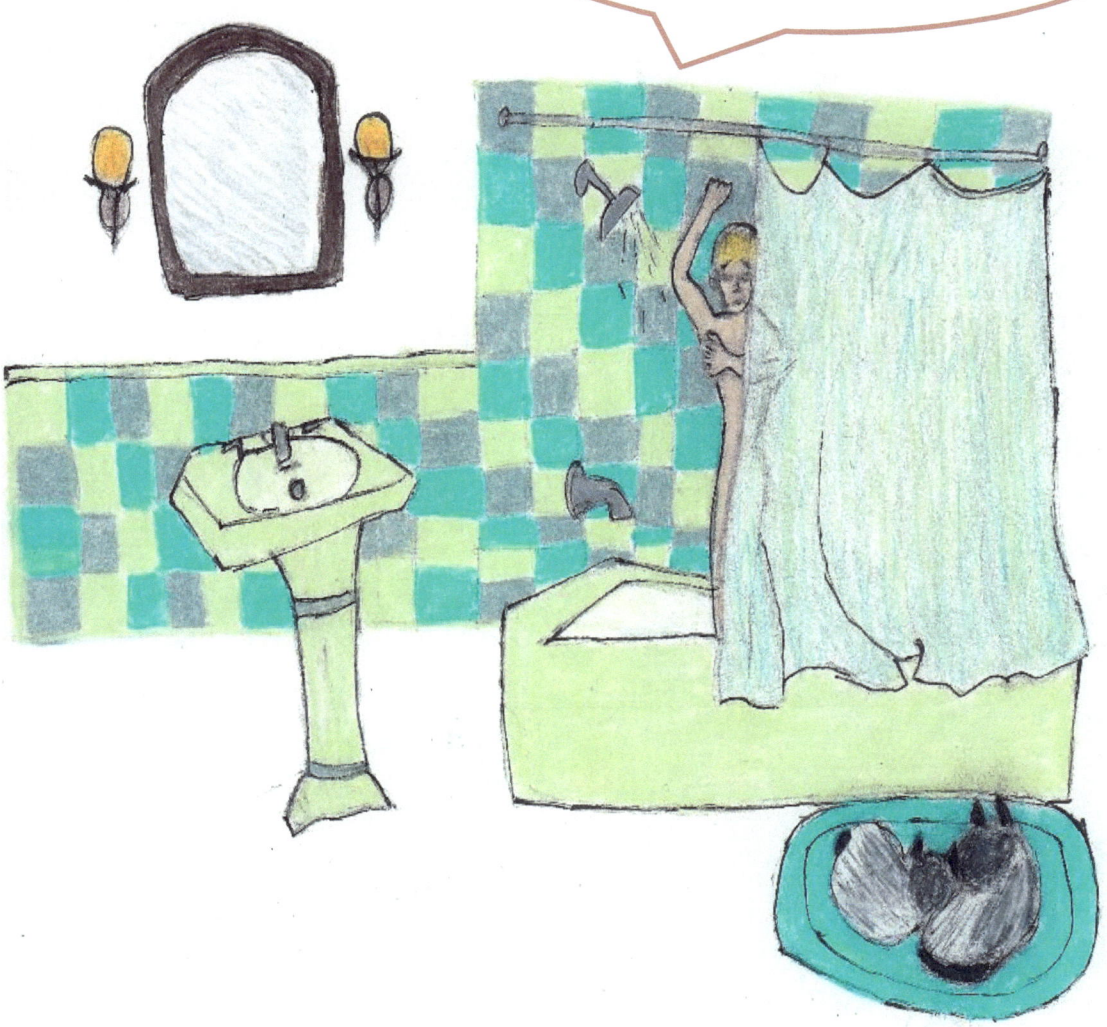

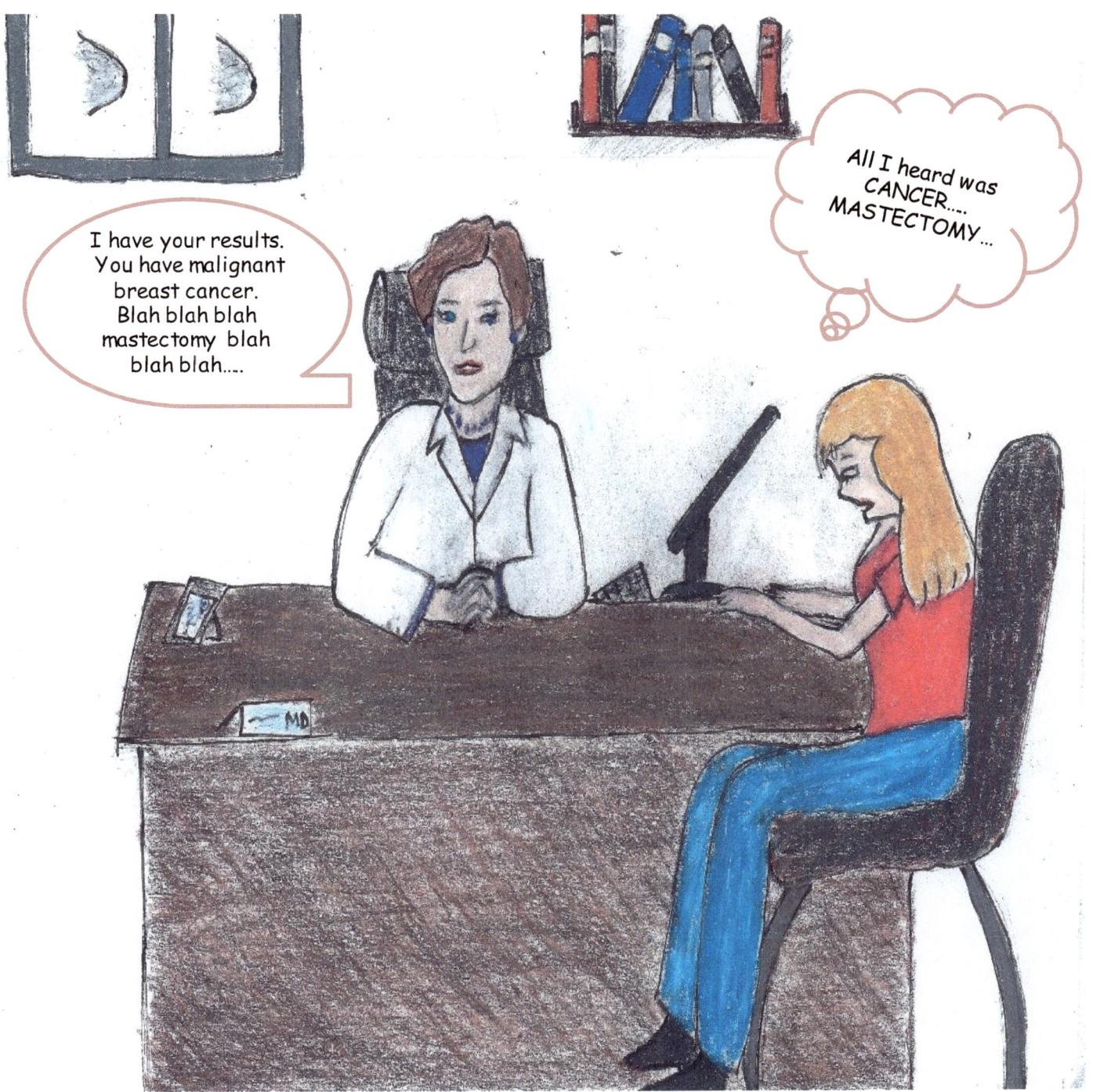

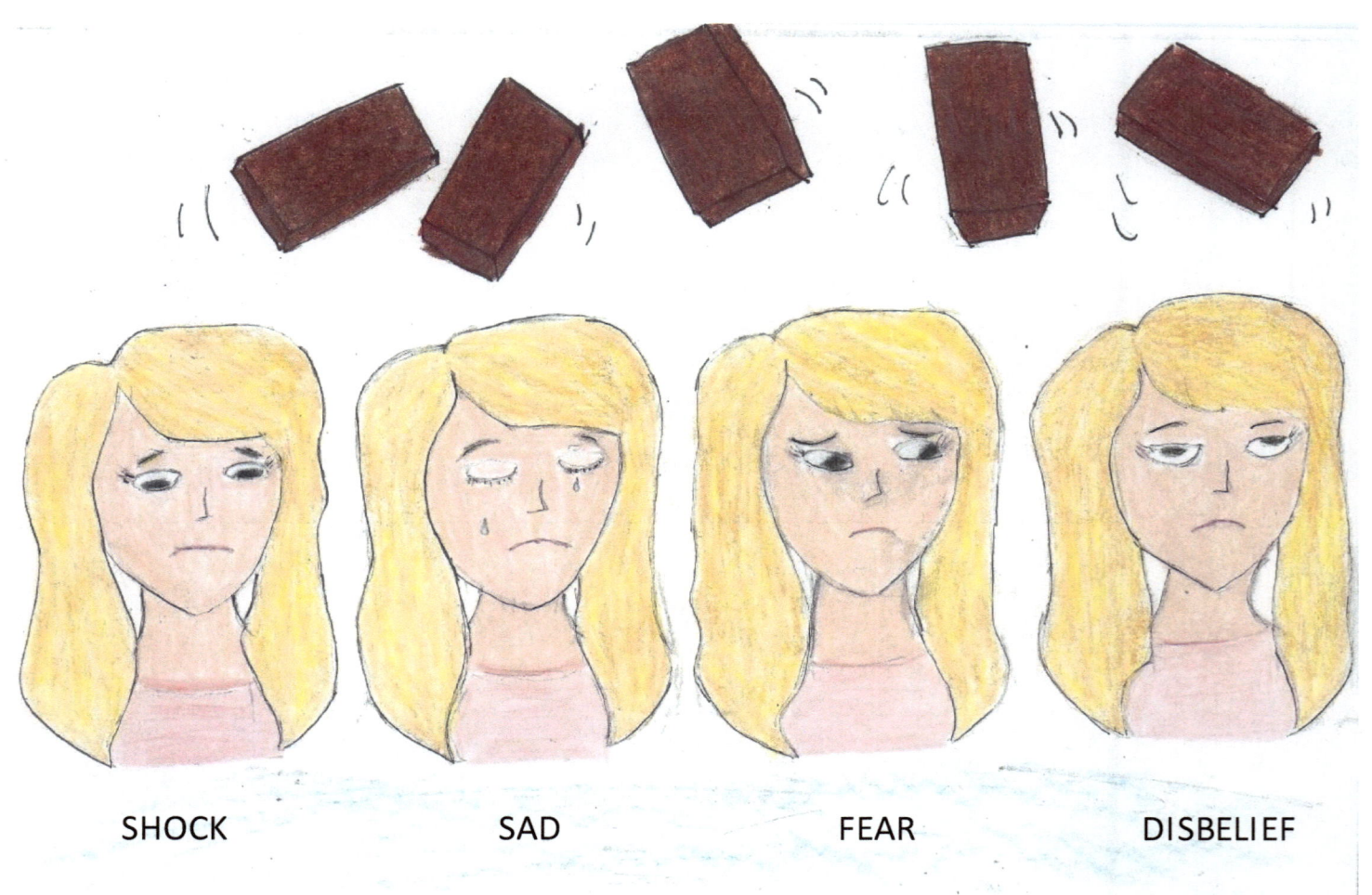

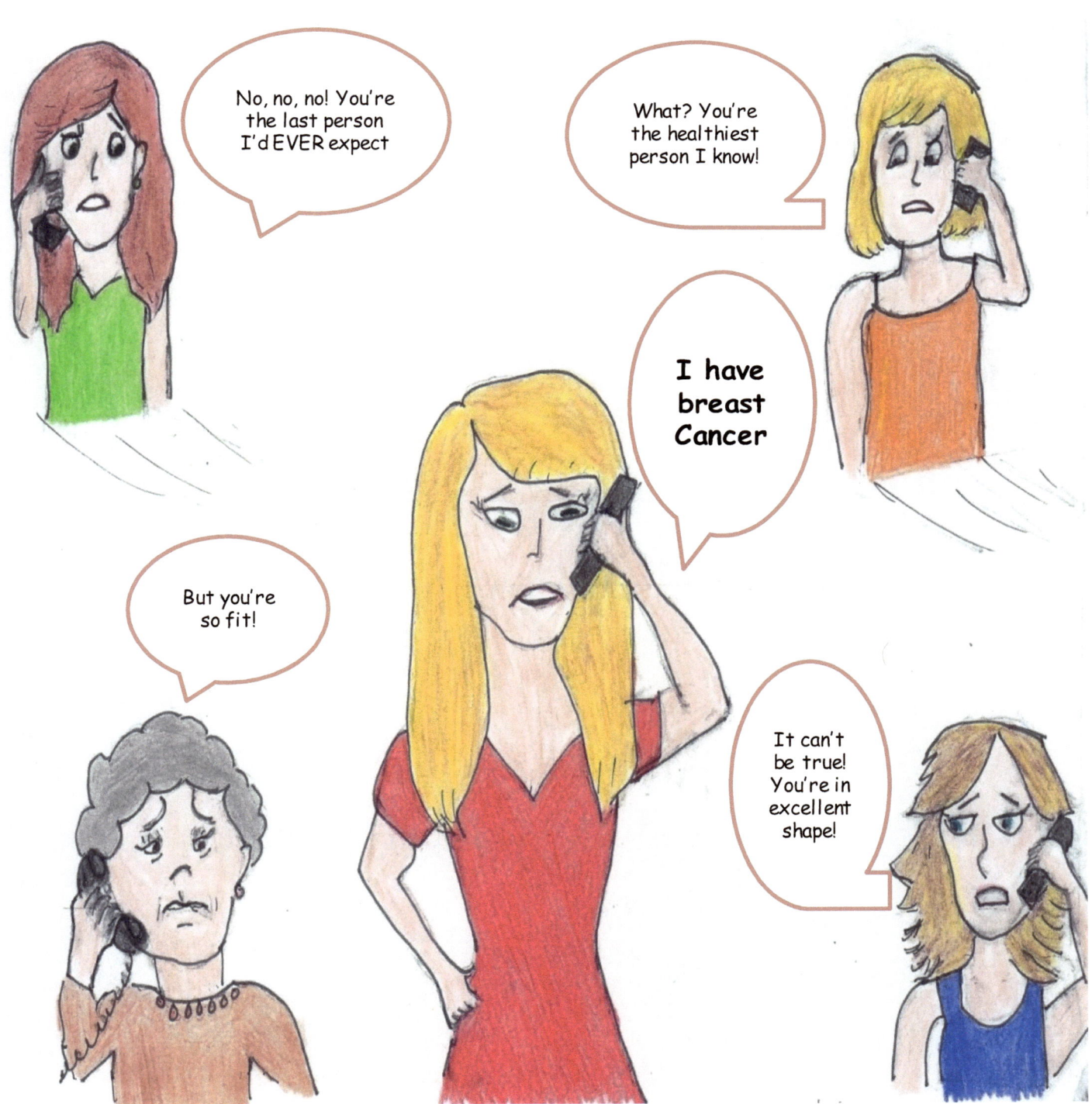

"My secret, private ritual. Good bye (sniff, sniff) beautiful body part, as I look at you for the last time."

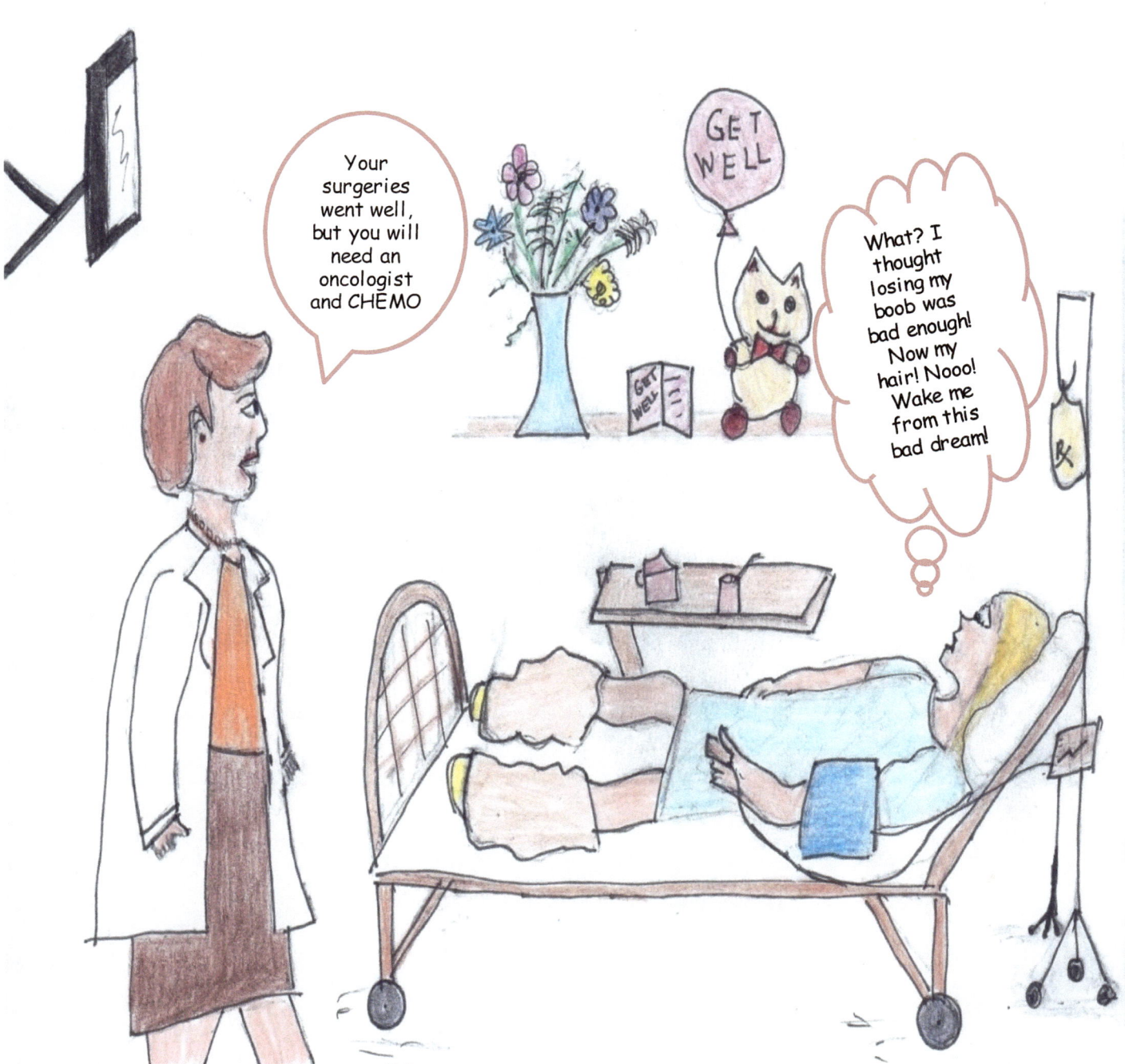

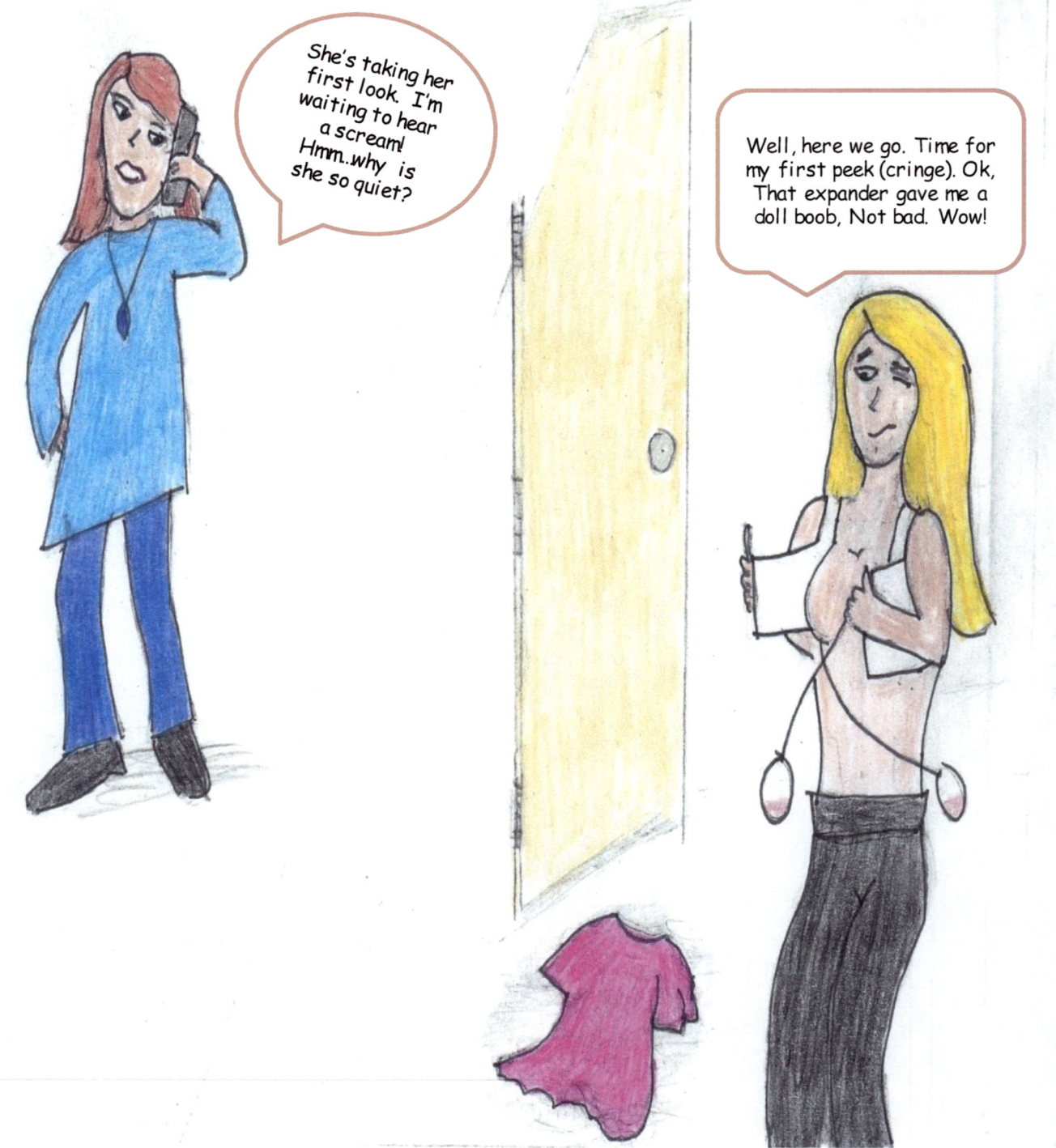

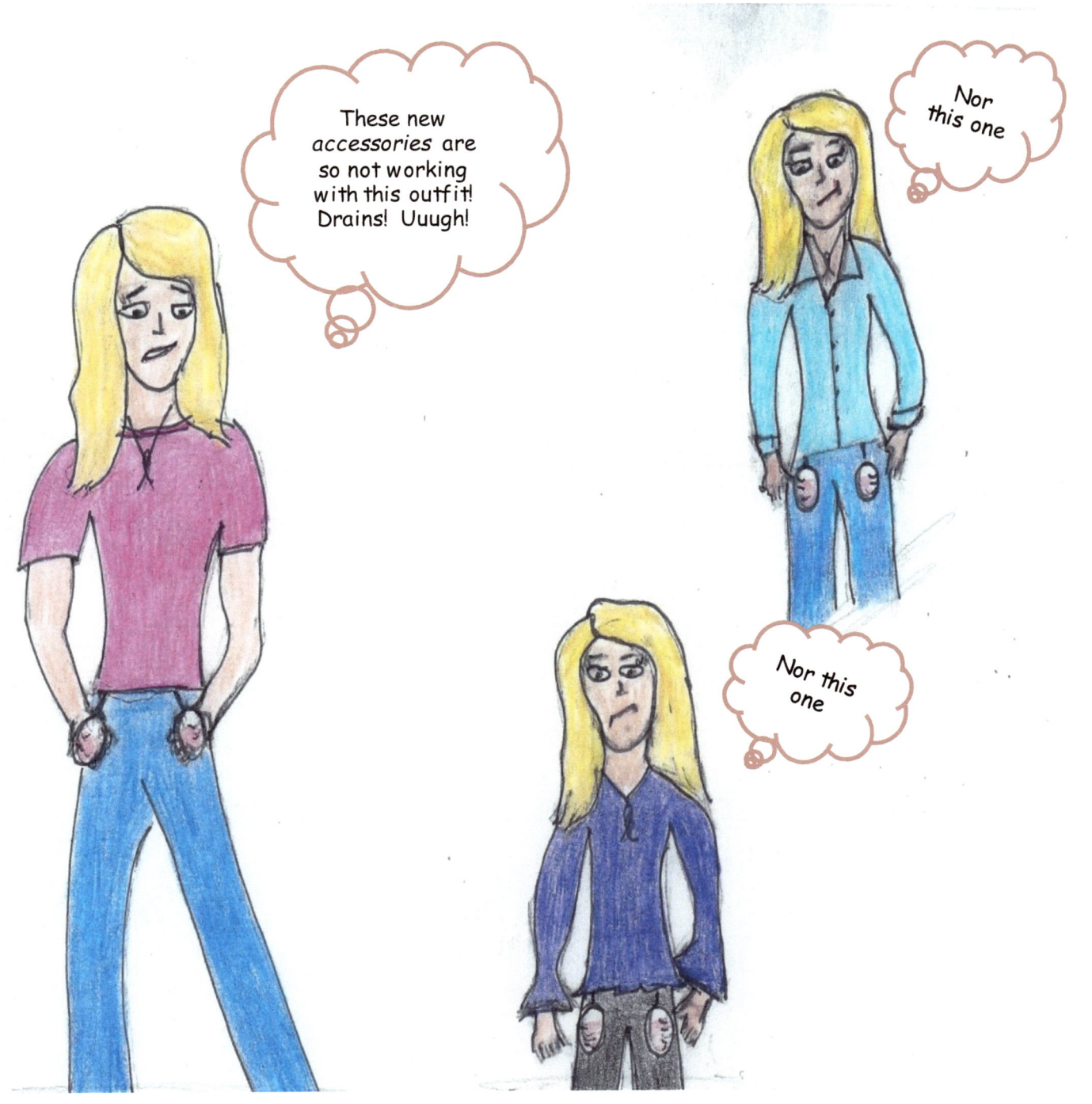

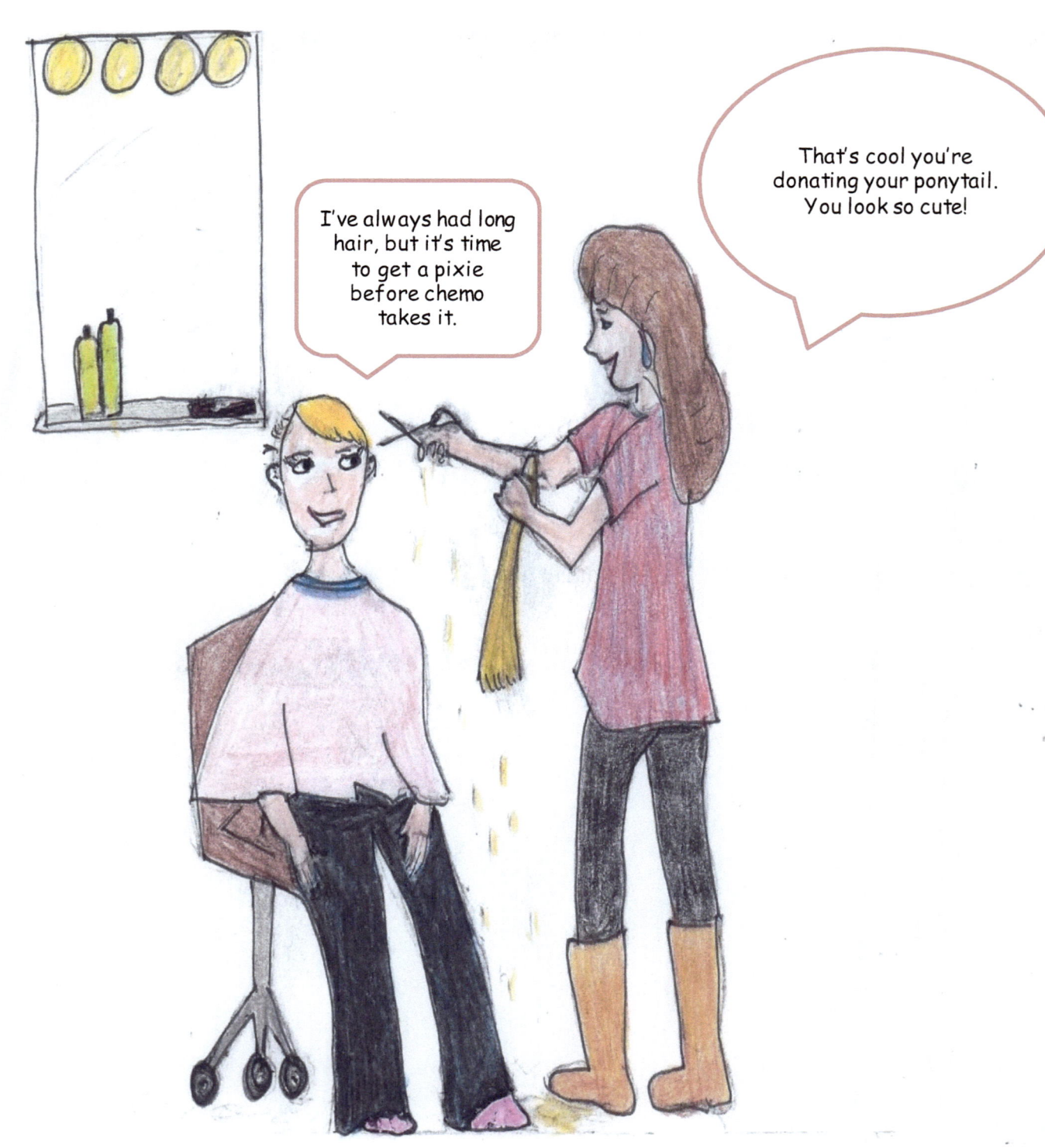

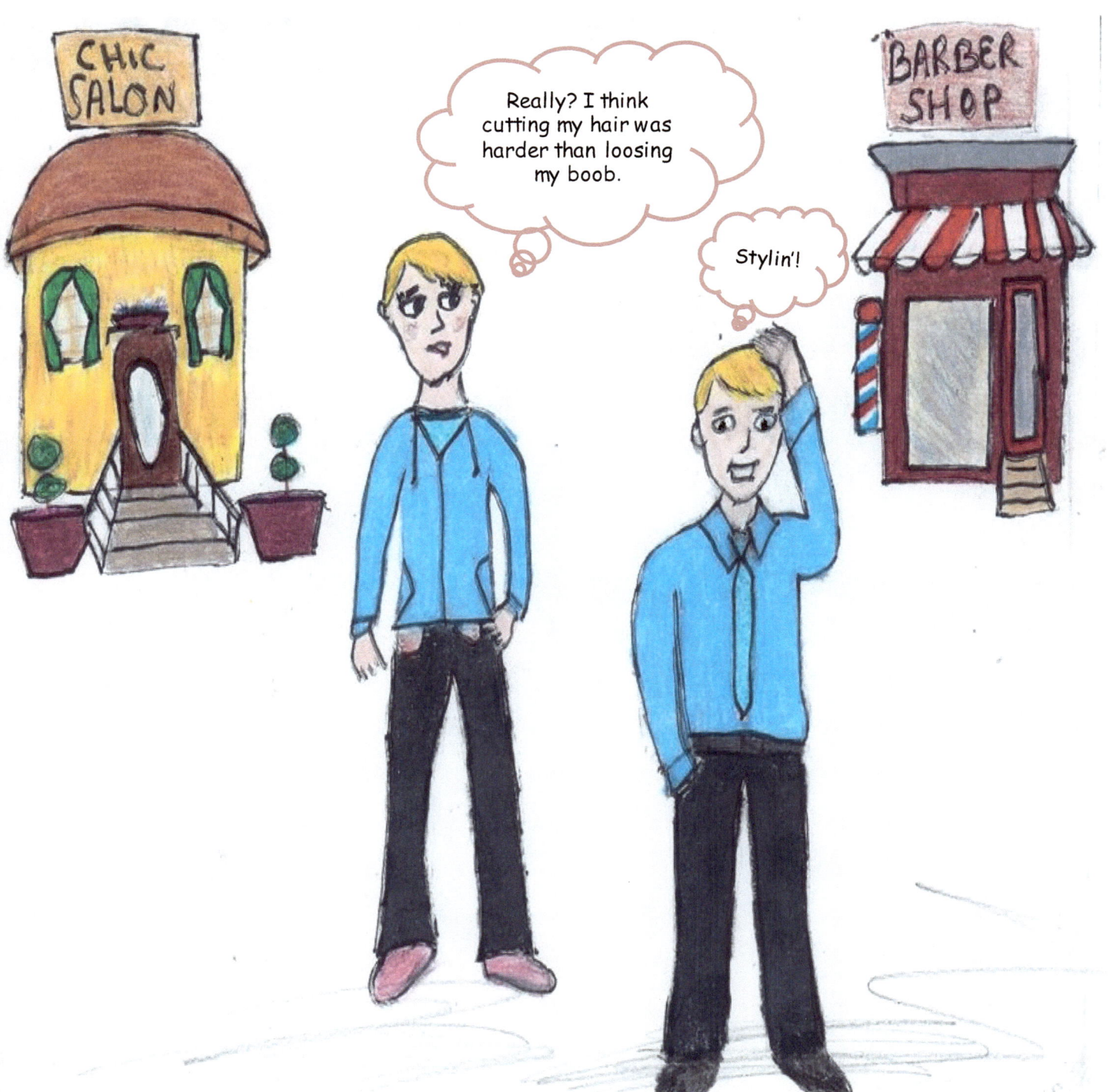

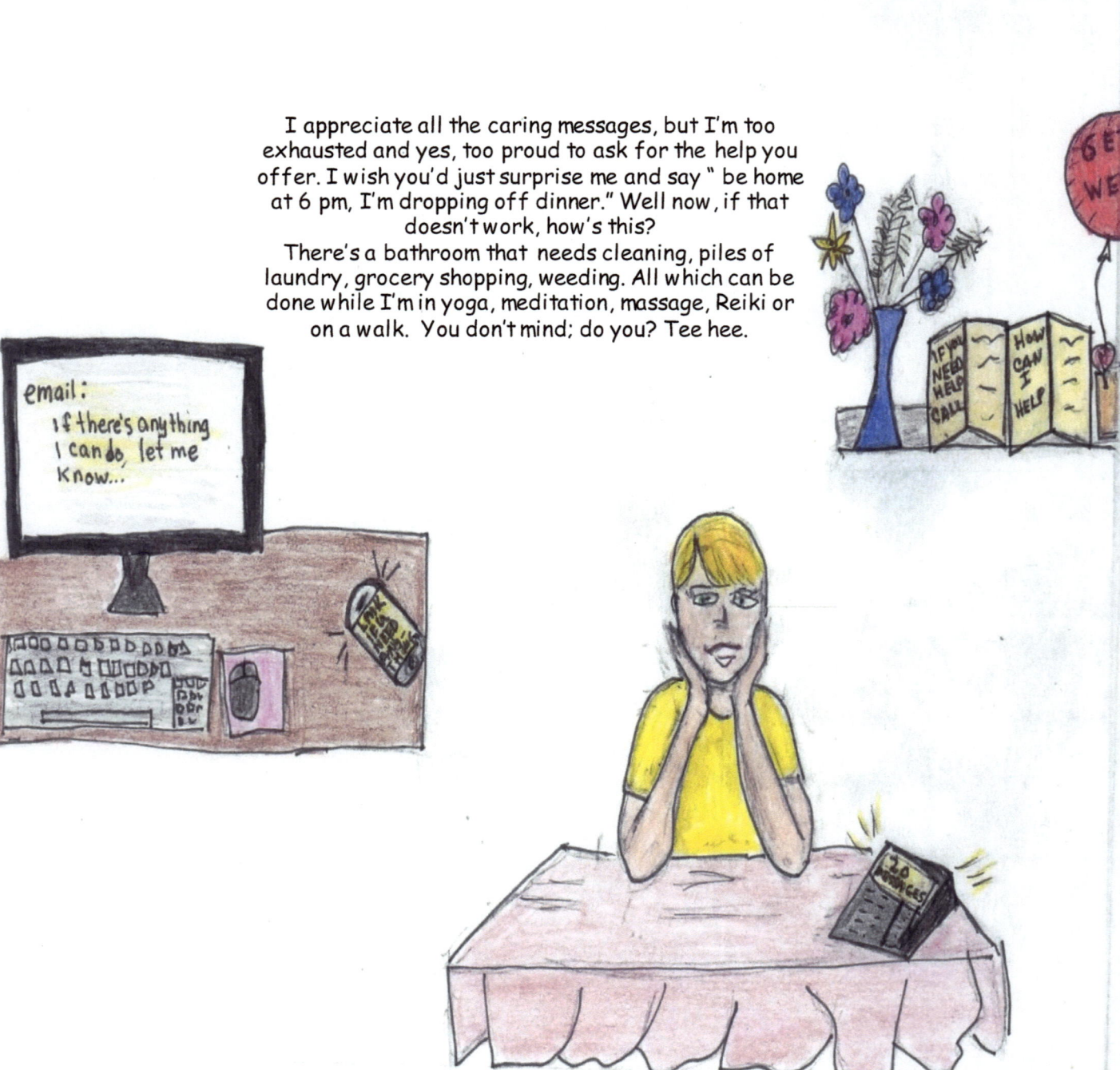

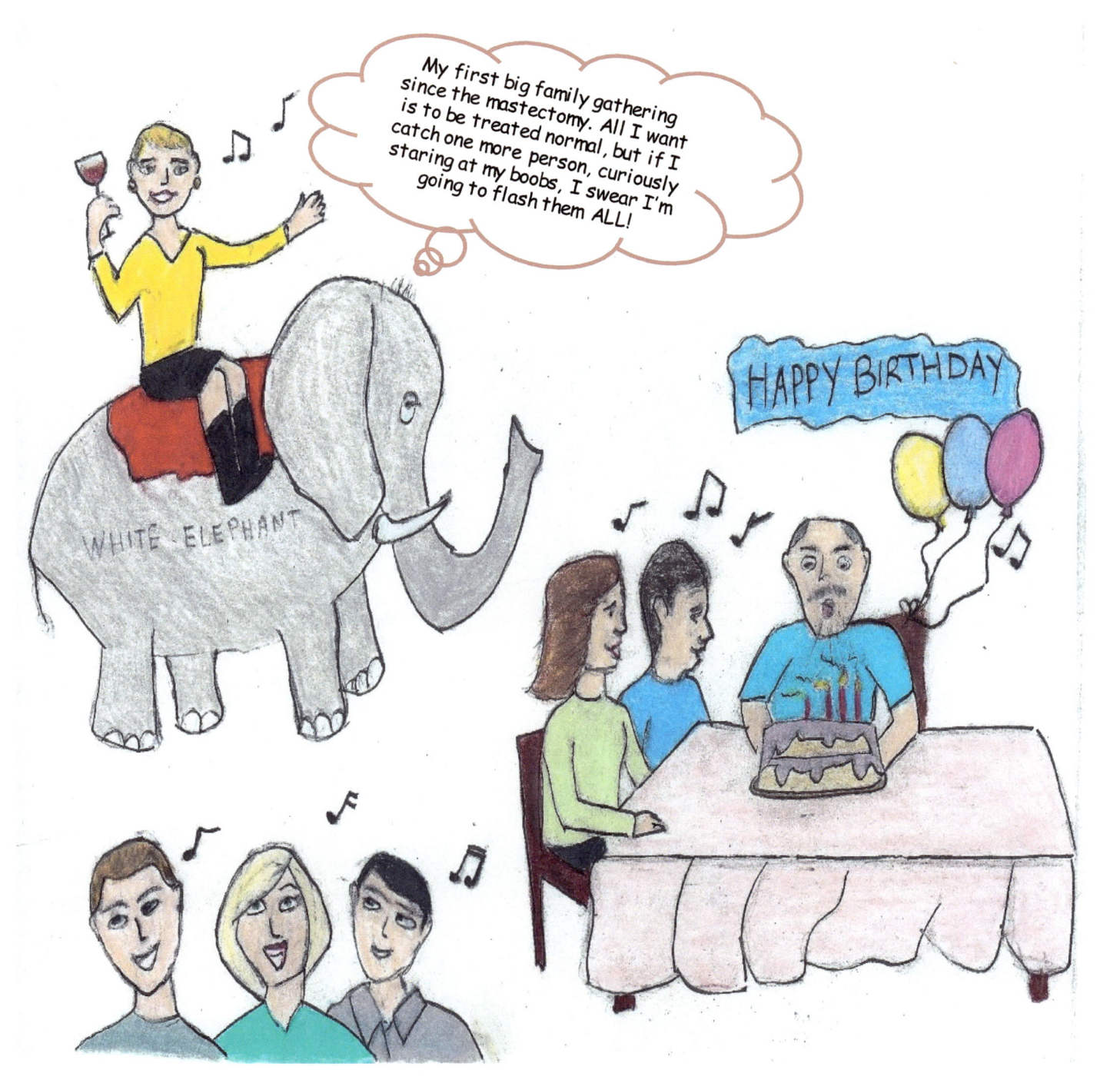

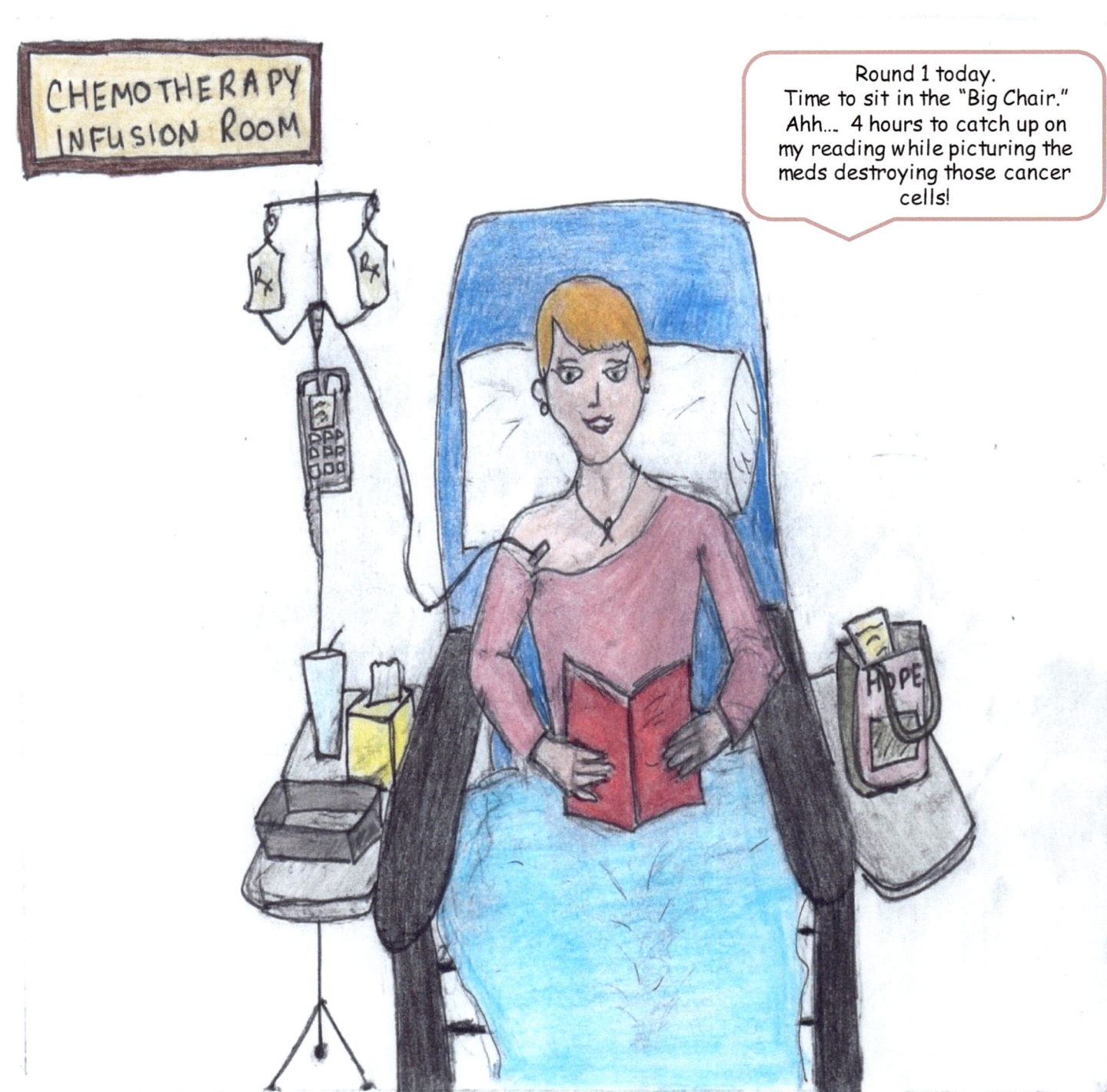

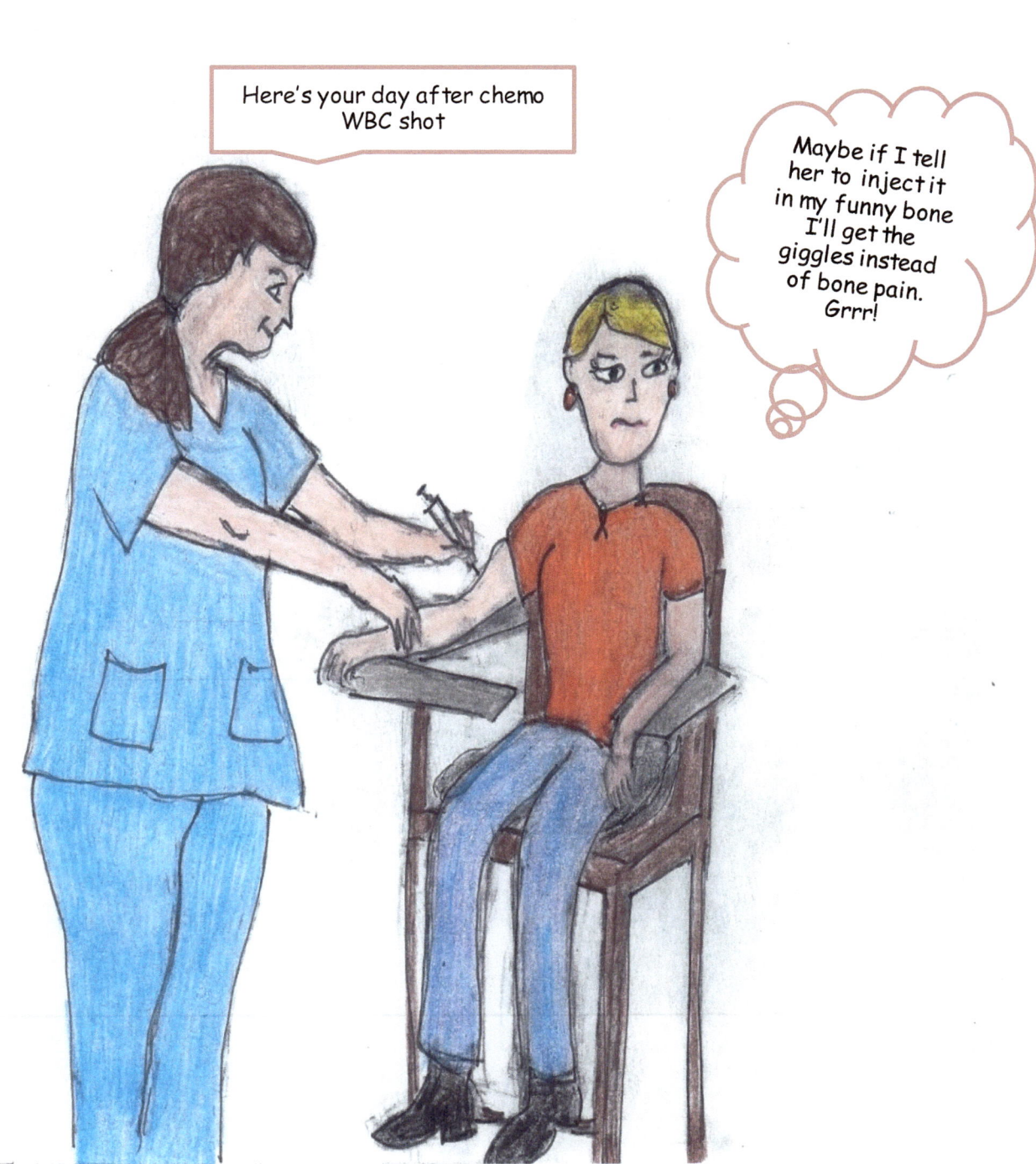

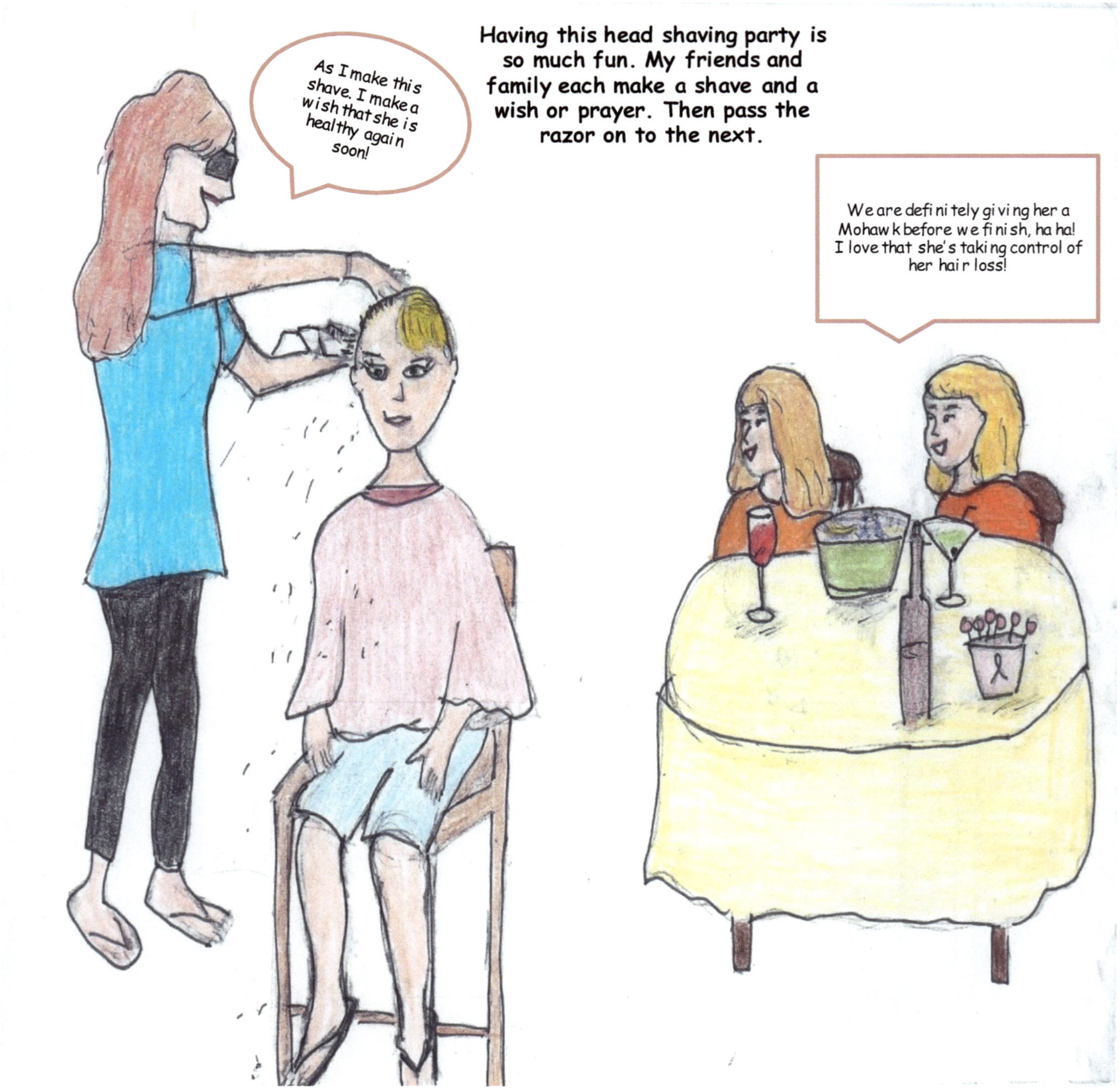

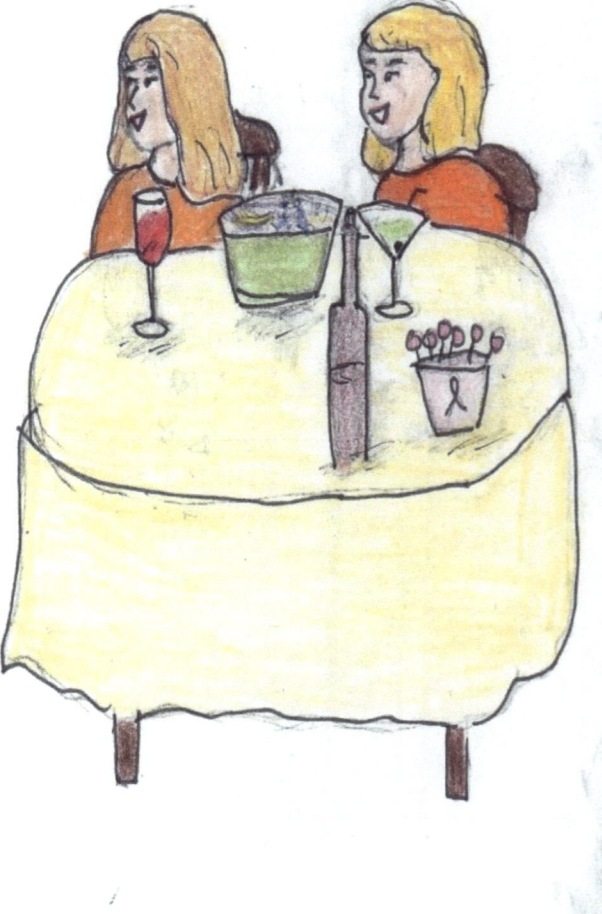

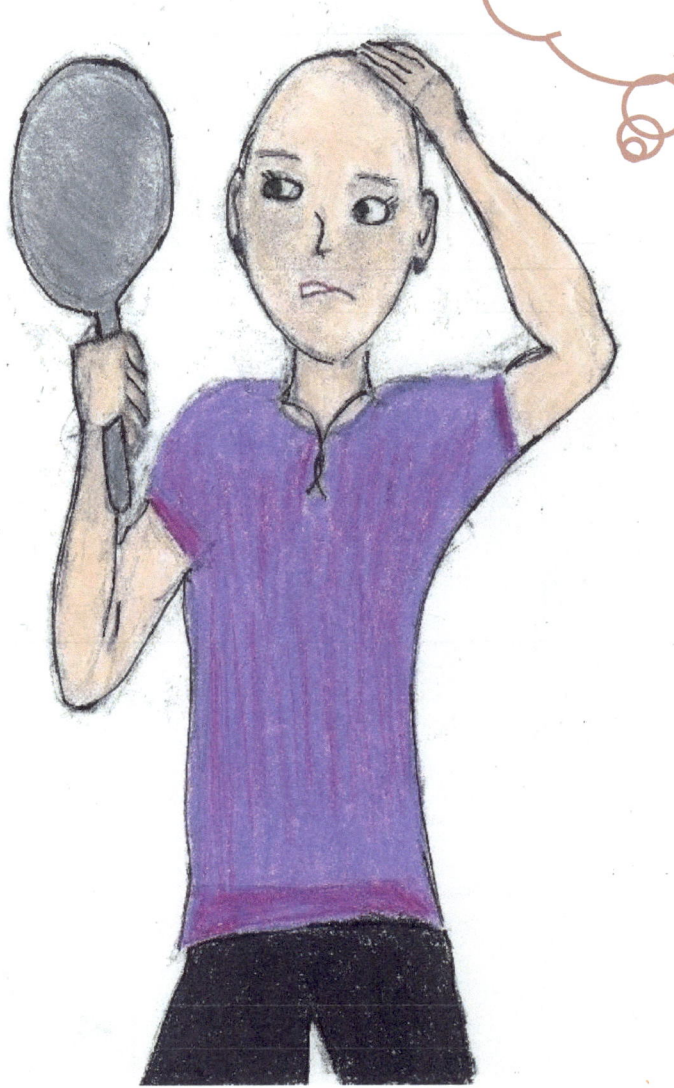

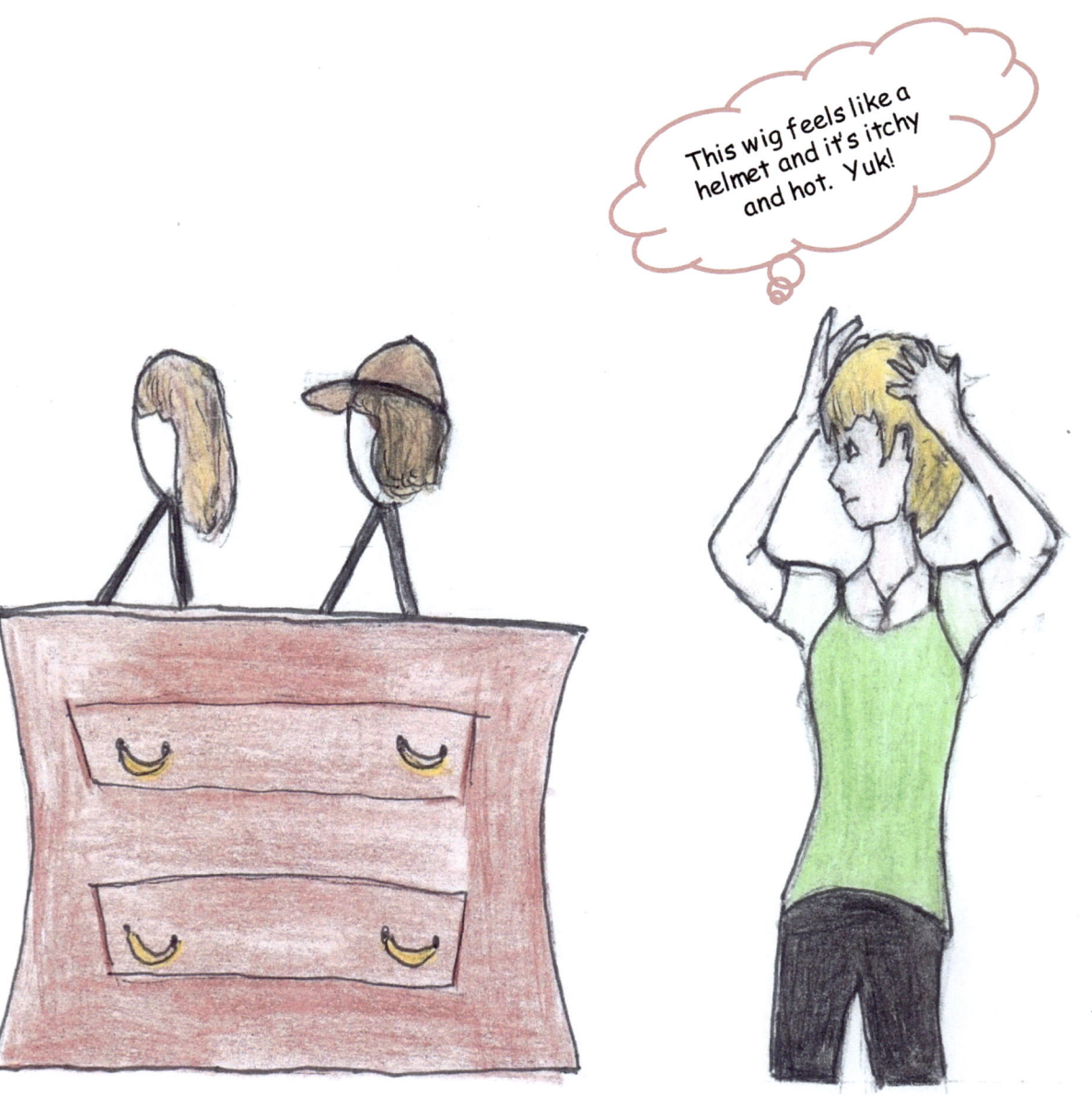

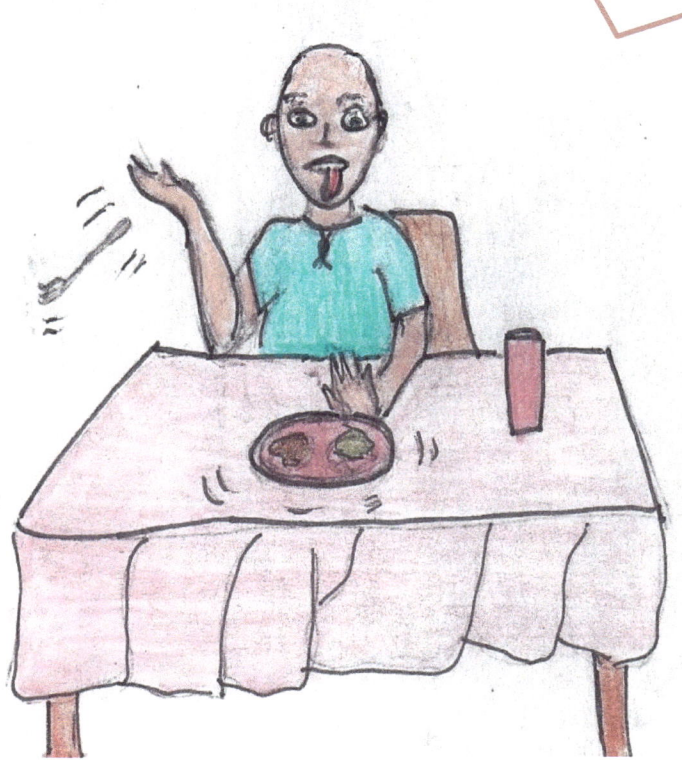

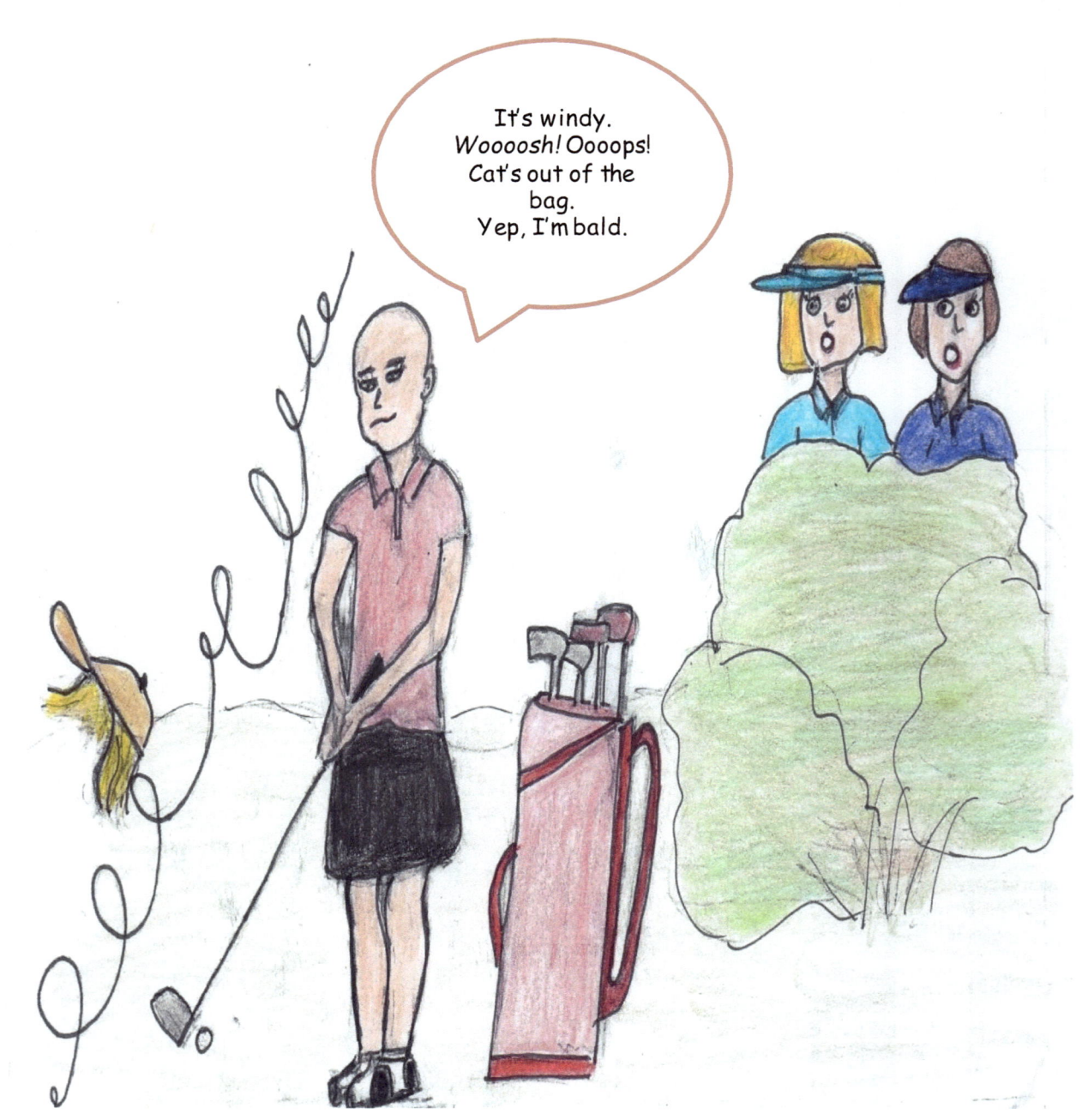

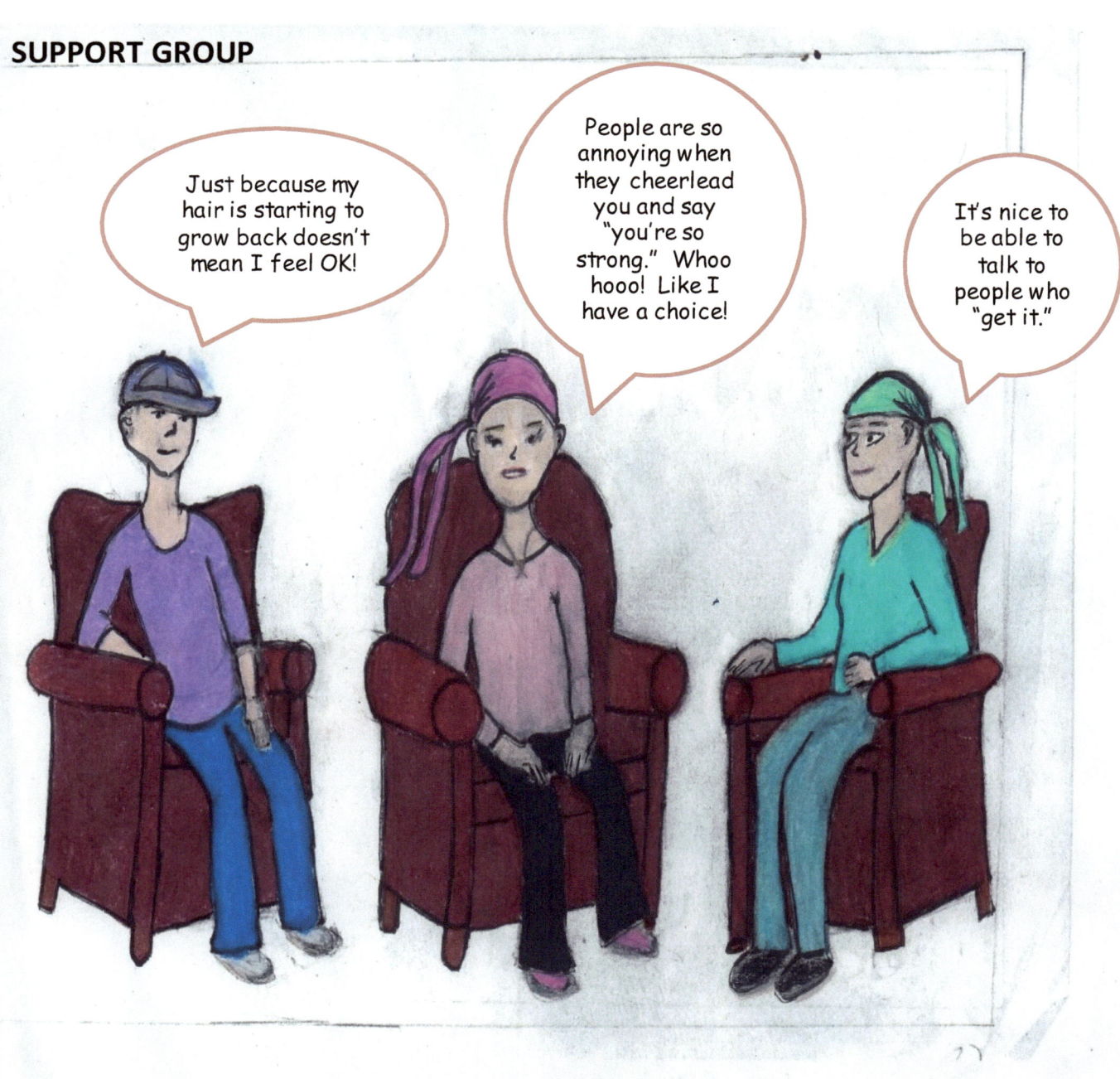

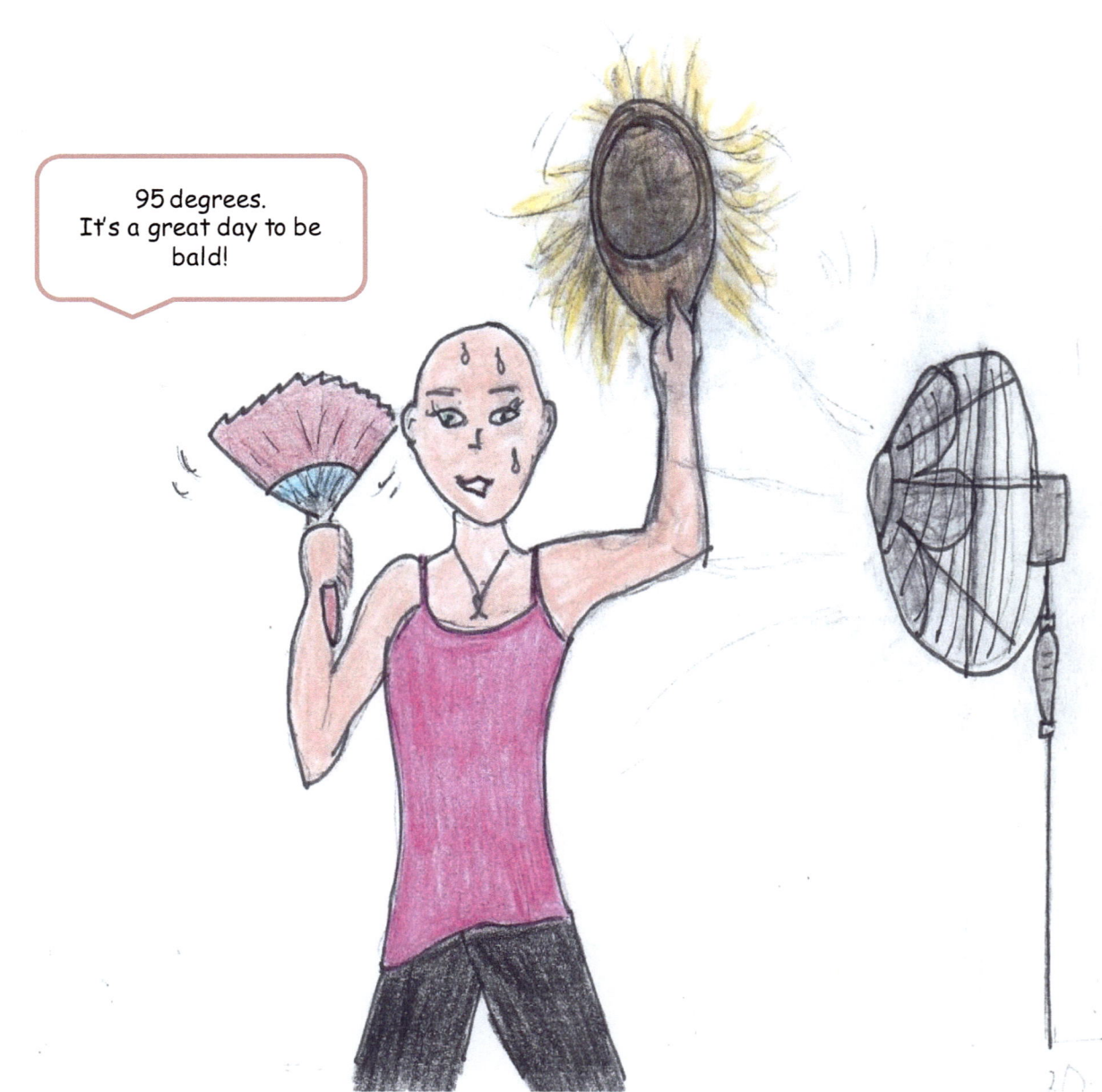

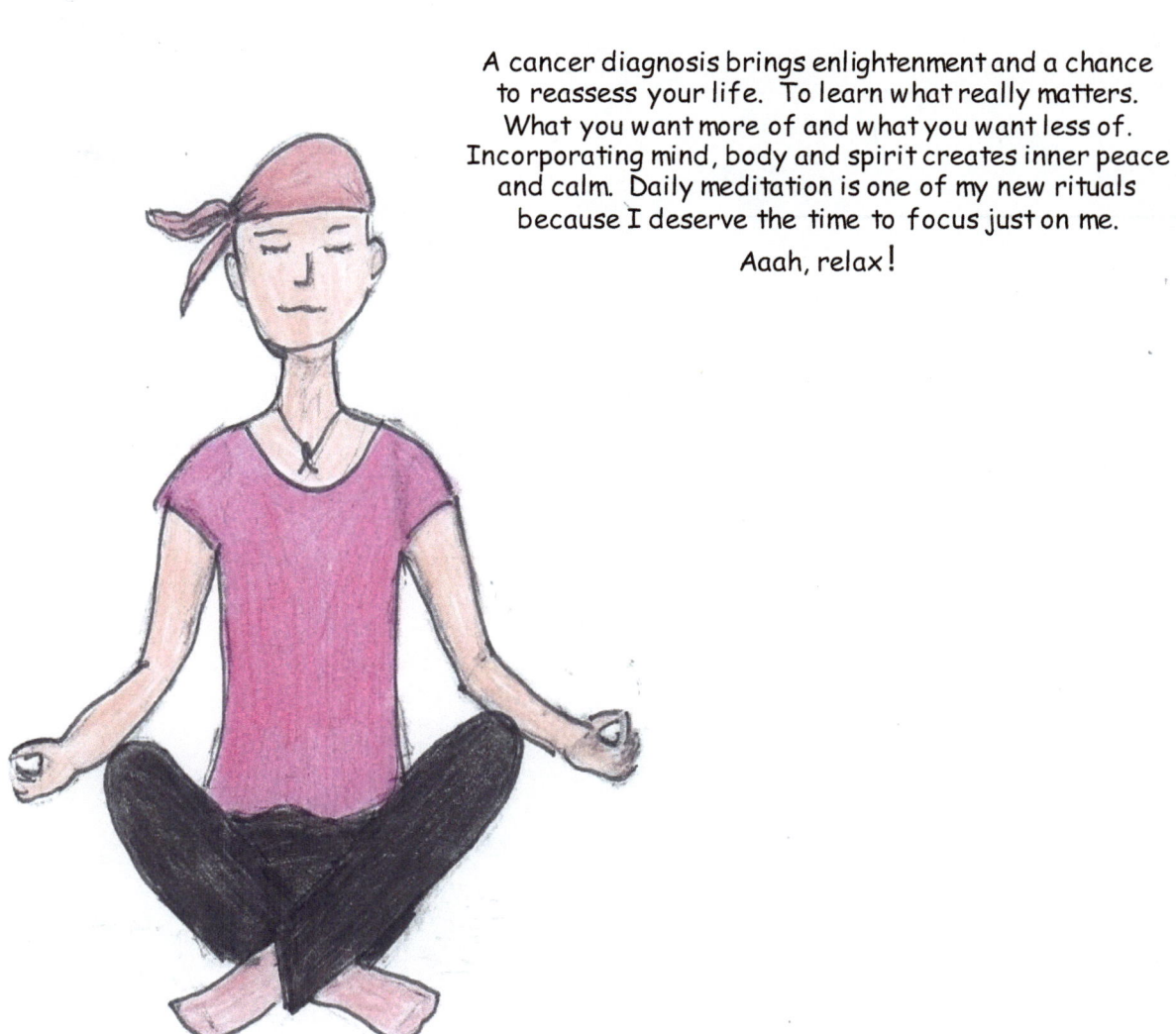

A cancer diagnosis brings enlightenment and a chance to reassess your life. To learn what really matters. What you want more of and what you want less of. Incorporating mind, body and spirit creates inner peace and calm. Daily meditation is one of my new rituals because I deserve the time to focus just on me.

Aaah, relax!

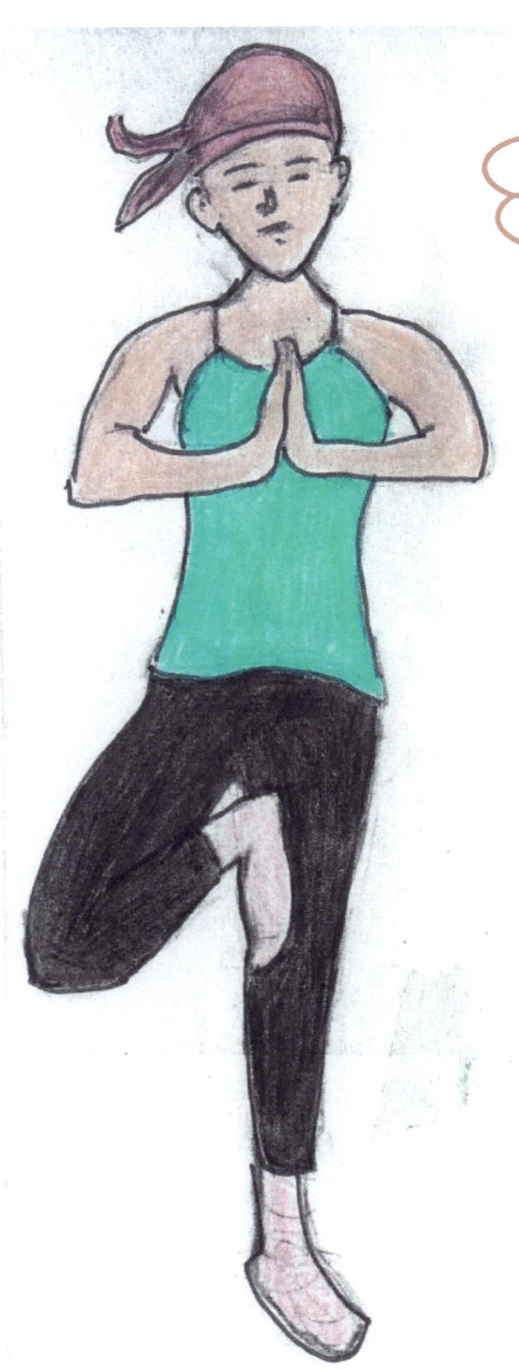

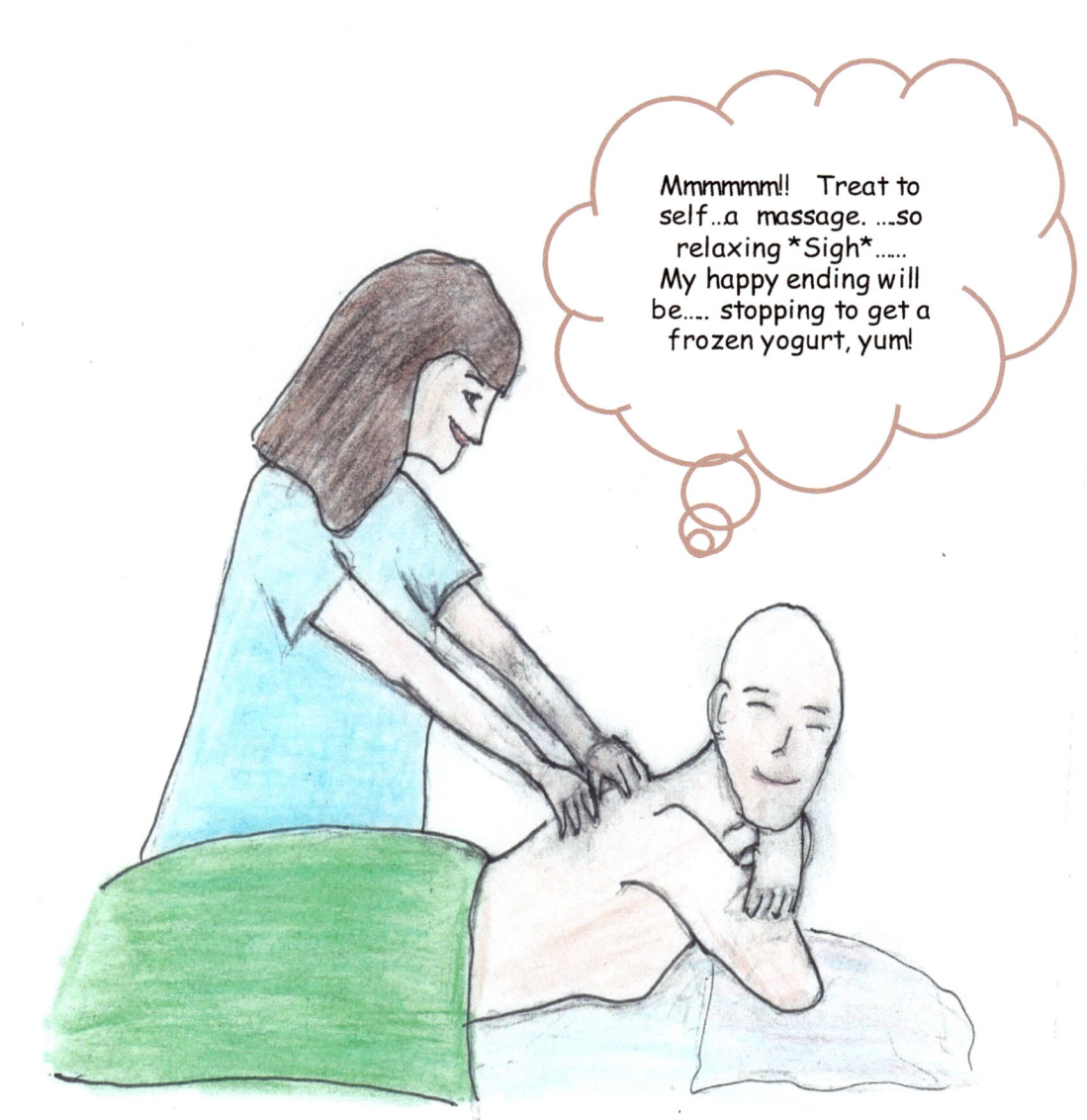

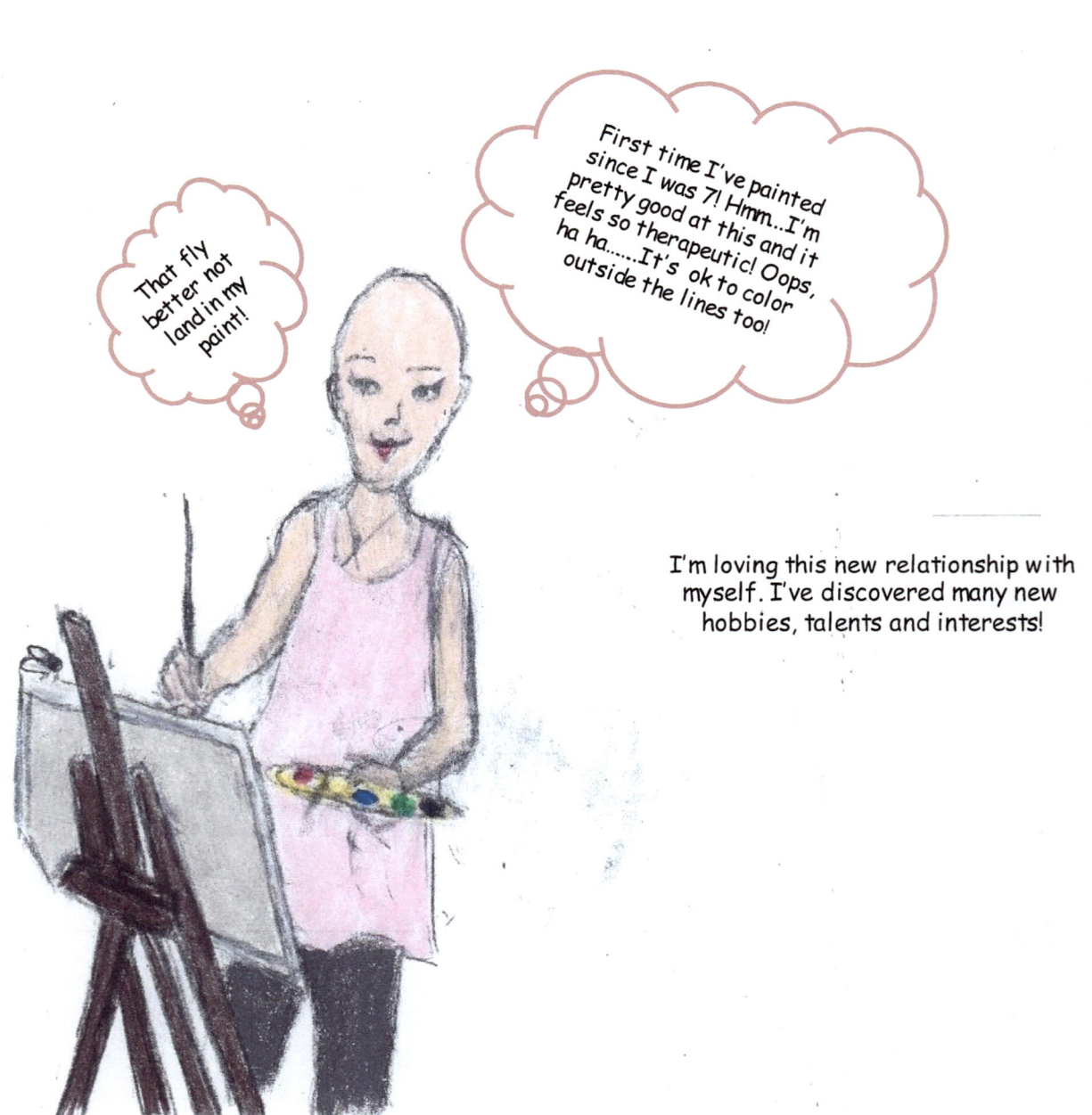

I'm loving this new relationship with myself. I've discovered many new hobbies, talents and interests!

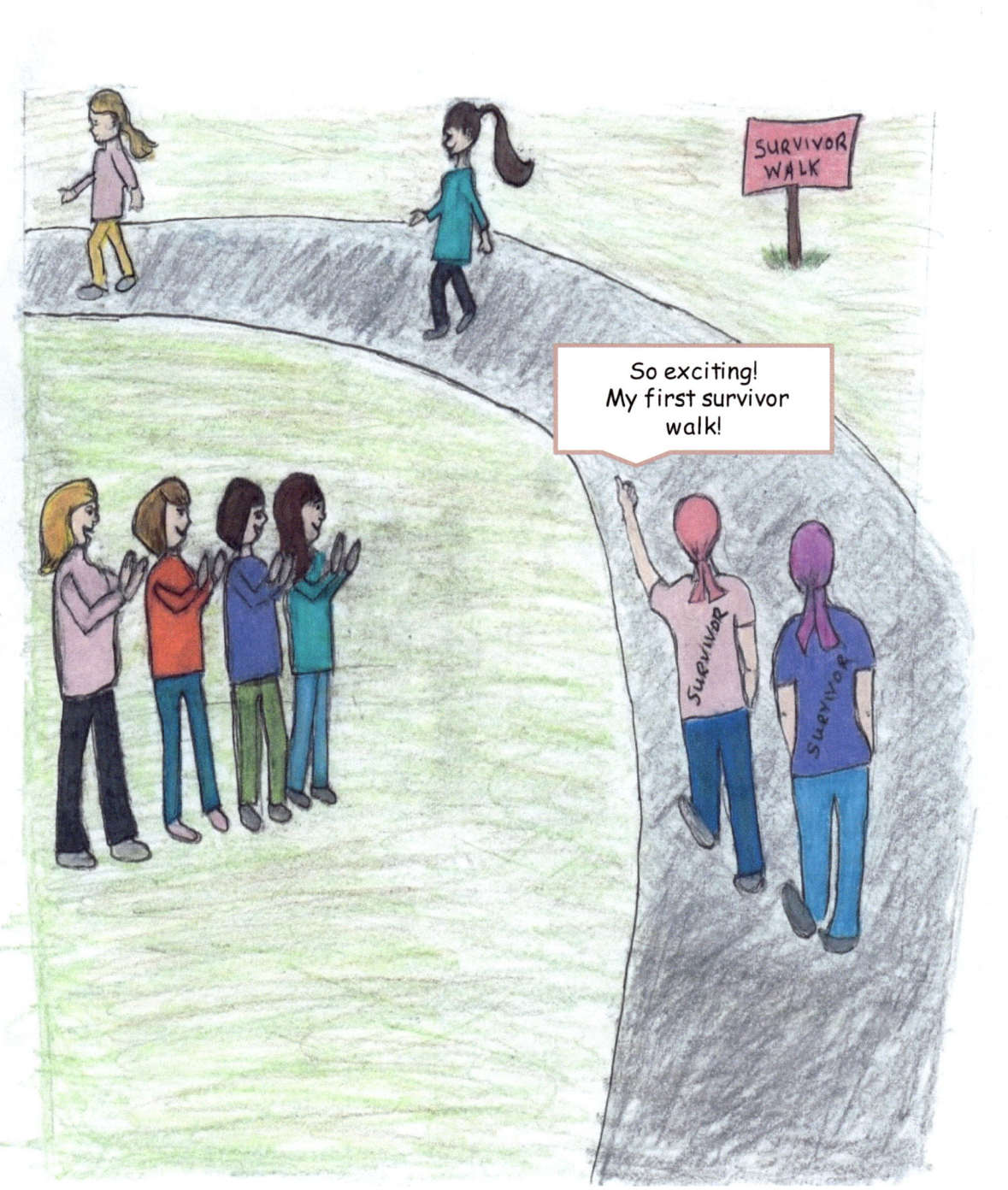

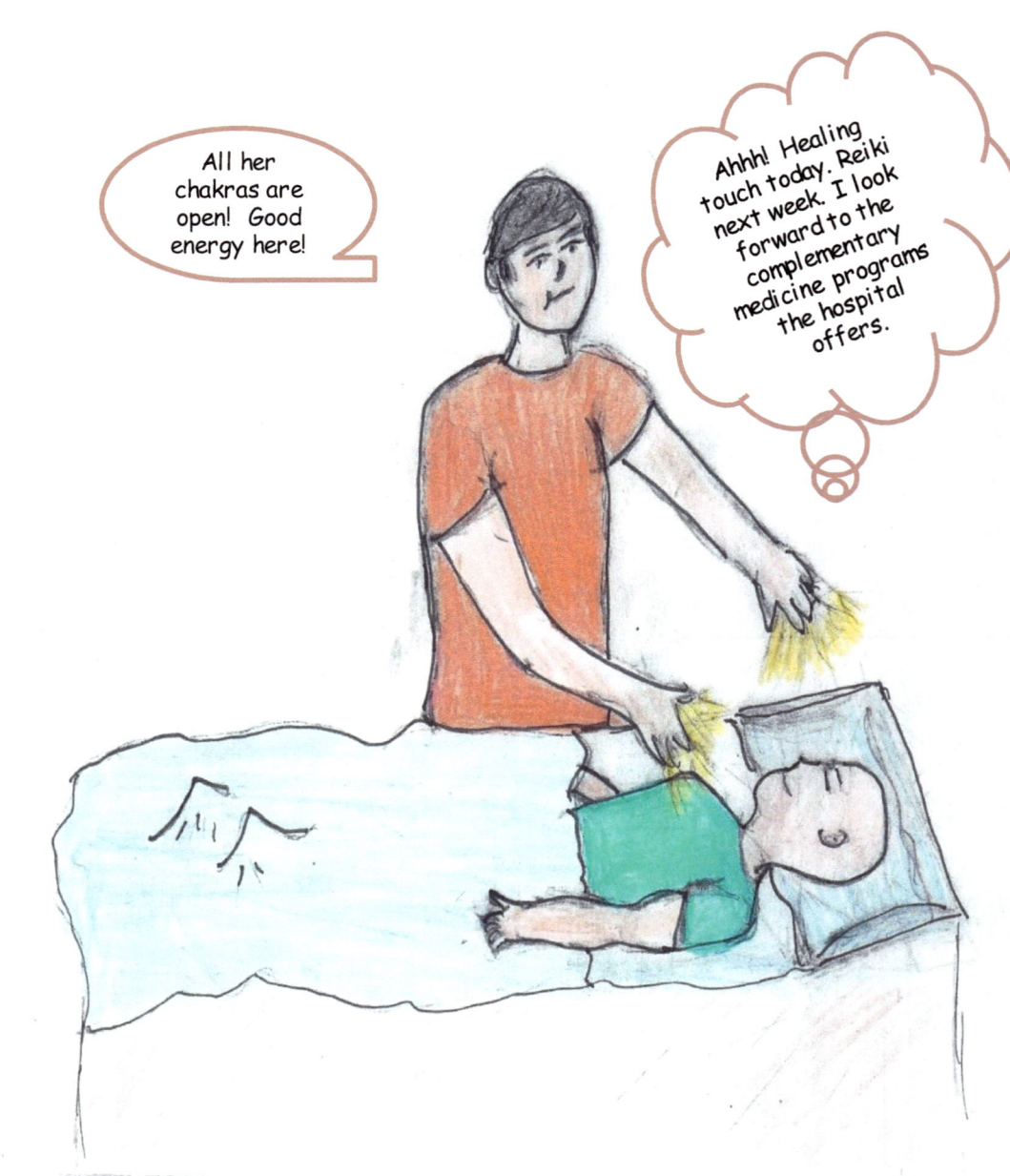

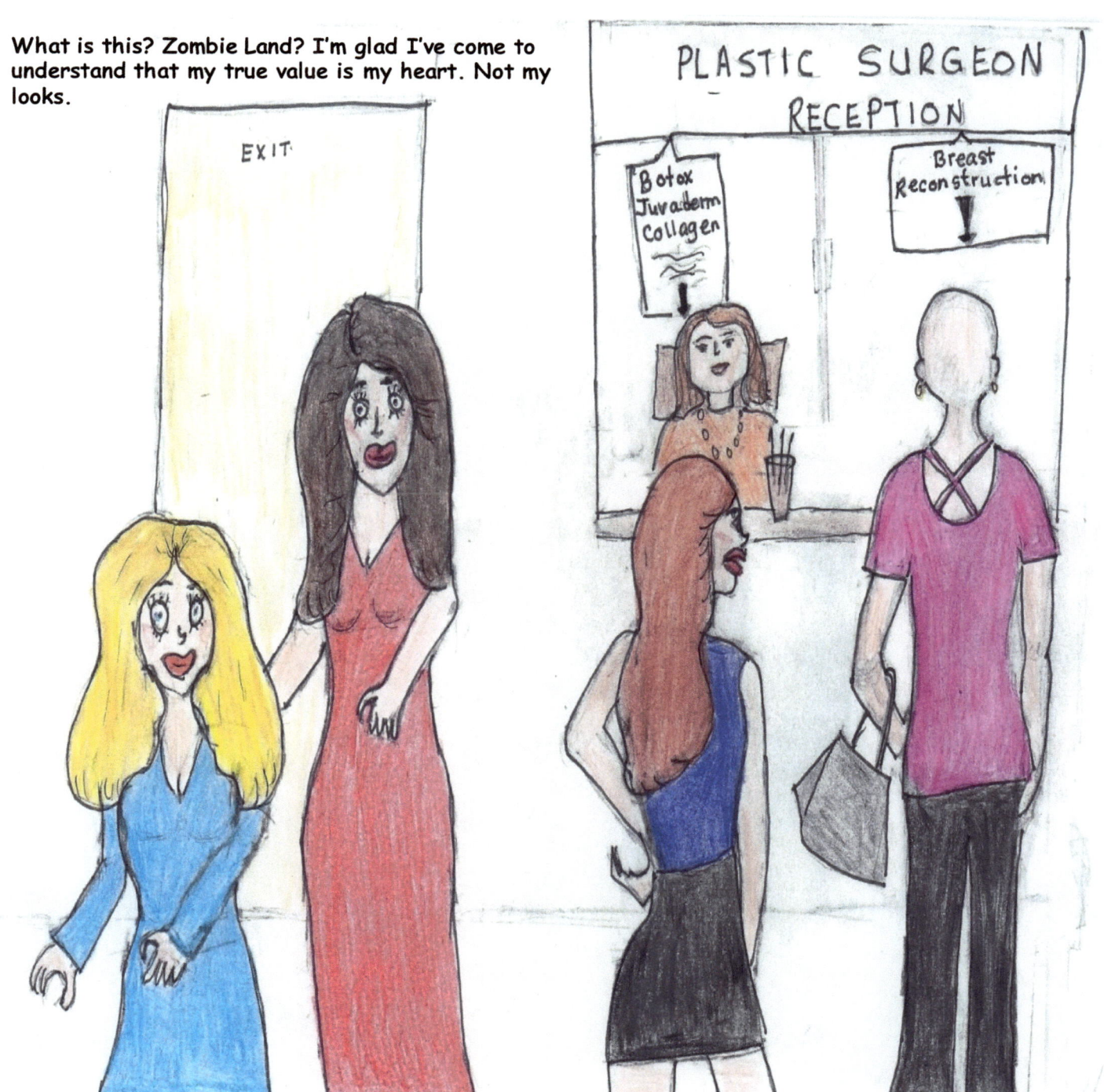

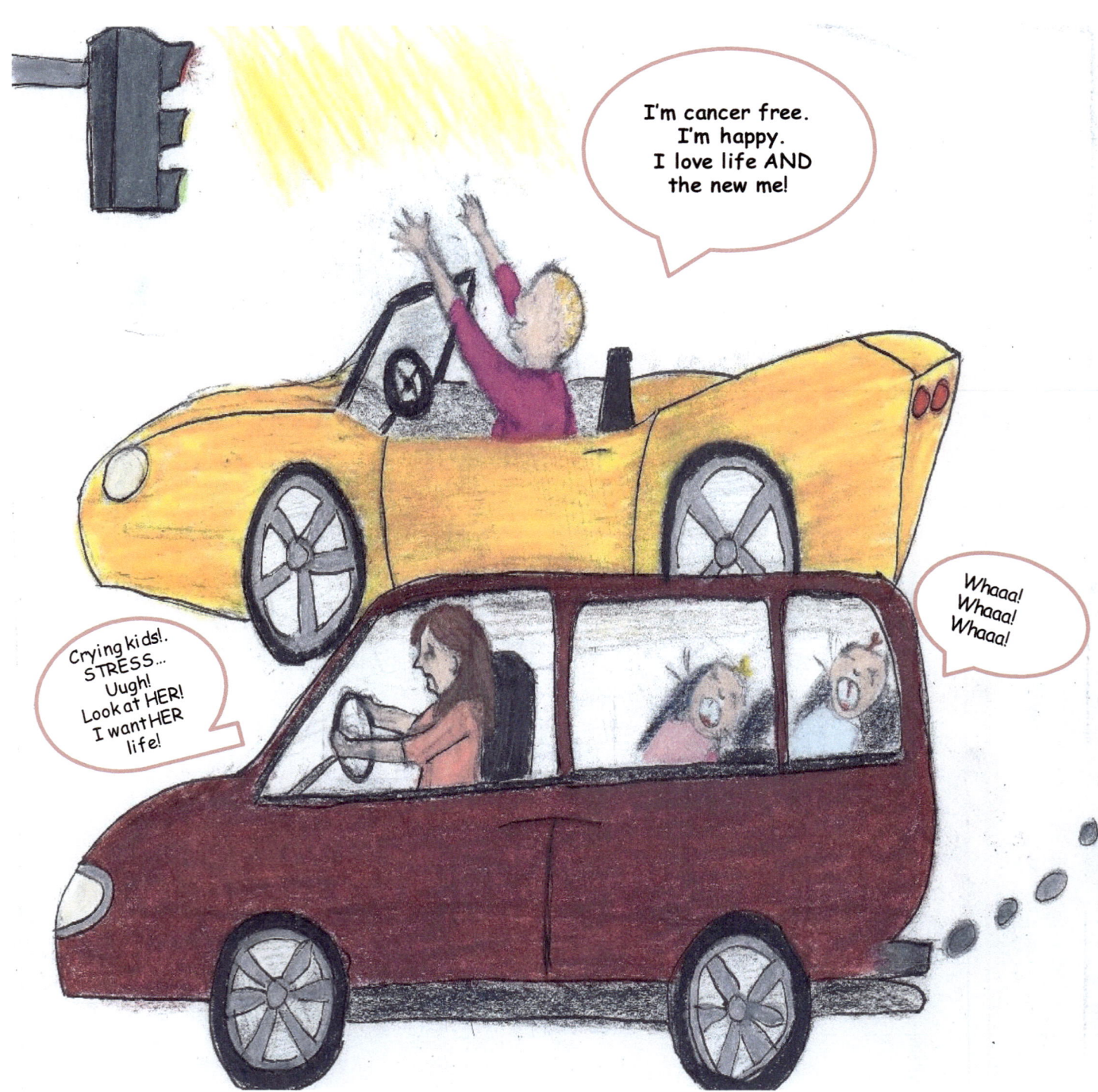

www.ingramcontent.com/pod-product-compliance
Lightning Source LLC
Chambersburg PA
CBHW040450220526
45473CB00004B/1587